P9-ELF-705

f **P**

the mind-beauty connection

9 Days to Reverse Stress Aging and Reveal More Youthful, Beautiful Skin

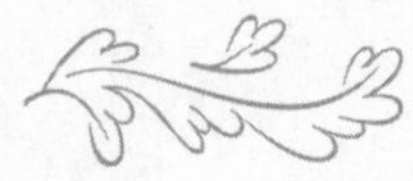

amy wechsler, md

Free Press
New York London Toronto Sydney

Note to Readers

This publication contains the opinions and ideas of its author. It is intended to provide helpful and informative material on the subjects addressed in the publication. It is sold with the understanding that the author and publisher are not engaged in rendering medical, health, or any other kind of personal professional services in the book. The reader should consult his or her medical, health, or other competent professional before adopting any of the suggestions in this book or drawing inferences from it.

The author and publisher specifically disclaim all responsibility for any liability, loss, or risk, personal or otherwise, which is incurred as a consequence, directly or indirectly, of the use and application of any of the contents of this book.

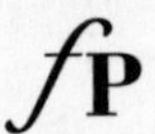

Free Press
A Division of Simon & Schuster, Inc.
1230 Avenue of the Americas
New York, NY 10020

Designed by Joel Avirom and Jason Snyder

Manufactured in the United States of America

ISBN-13: 978-1-4165-6257-3

For Zoe, Jaden, and Harry

contents

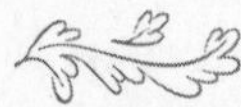

introduction

An End to Stress Age

How old do you look? How old do you *think* you look? If a simple Q&A test in front of the mirror could tell you what your physical age is—regardless of your chronological age—what do you think it would reveal? You are about to find out. In the very first chapter, you're going to take three quizzes, one of which is revolutionary. Designed by RealAge, the SkinAge test will tell you exactly how old you really look. It will mark your starting point for a step-by-step program outlined in this book that will transform you from the inside out, and it will get everyone to notice.

If you have been frustrated or unhappy with your appearance—whether you are twenty-two or sixty-two—then this is the book for you. Chances are, you picked up this book for a reason. Maybe it's the unprecedented acne, the deep lines and shallow crinkles, the lack of a healthy glow, the thinning hair and brittle nails, the extra ten pounds you didn't have a year ago, or perhaps it's the accelerated aging in general that is evident everywhere you look when you step in front of a mirror. And maybe you avoid the mirror at all costs now. No matter what your personal issues are with your appearance, I am here to show you how to change all that. After all, loving the skin you are in is essential to personal well-being. In fact, in my practice, how you look is a vital sign of health.

There is so much you can do with great results without taking radical action or going under a knife. My approach is uncomplicated, effective, and empowering. No frills. No gimmicks. You'll be shocked to learn my easy daily practices that can bring out radiant, natural beauty. And for you busy moms who feel as though you are not allowed to look fabulous, listen up. I'm a mom, too, and I can't express how important it is to nurture yourself with today's cutting-edge strategies to maximize health and, of course, beauty. Your whole family will benefit.

When RealAge approached me to do a book, I was thrilled at the opportunity to get the message out about what it takes to stay looking and feeling as vibrant as possible, with a focus on the very skin that wraps us up so wonderfully. Some people will stop at nothing to find the secrets to maintaining their youthful looks and heightening their attractiveness, and throw thousands of dollars at the beauty industry. If only they knew that the secret is learning one powerful principle, and following a plan that abides by it.

Contrary to popular belief, skin is not just the passive barrier that we used to think it was. It's a very active organ. The mind and other organs communicate with each other, both directly through nerves and indirectly through chemical messengers.

This principle is the mind-beauty connection, and it lies at the heart of achieving the most beautiful skin (and, I might add, body) possible. On a most basic level, the mind-beauty connection is about the powerful force that exists between our inner minds and outer appearances, which is based on proven biochemistry. Astonishing new science is revealing just how our minds affect how well, and how fast, we age physically. This includes not only how we think and our behavior, but also how we cope with the madness of modern life, and how we preserve our bodies' self-healing and inherent beautification capabilities. What's more, scientists continue to uncover incredible insights into how our skin, in addition to our brains, is also an extraordinary command center for communication, and is able to effect change in our inner bodies and outer appearance in ways we never thought possible before.

the sensitive and simple approach

This book will inspire you to make a few small shifts in how you take care of yourself with practical and doable recommendations. I'm not here to sell you expensive products, or tell you to use anything that hasn't been clinically proven to work *on people*. You see, so many of the lotions, potions, and so-called must-haves that line the drugstores' shelves and beauty counters overclaim and underperform. Promising laboratory studies don't always translate into real-world effectiveness in humans. I will not only dispel myths in the beauty-market circles, but I will also give you sound advice to help you distinguish the hype from the truly helpful. I will state plainly what you can do starting today to improve your appearance (and strengthen your self-confidence, too!) without falling prey to great advertising. And for those who do choose to explore more aggressive procedures like Botox and resurfacing, I'll give you the guidance to find the right solution for you, your wallet, and your peace of mind.

Premature aging and adult acne are the two most common skin problems I see, and I often find that I have to get to the bottom of exhaustion or emotional issues in order to treat these symptoms of modern life. There are plenty of combination strategies that can help reverse the effects of tension and time. I was a psychiatrist for seven years before I became board certified in dermatology and switched specialties. I put my old hat on every day to untangle the psychological from the physical and find sensitive, simple, solutions for both.

the front line of defense

My experience in psychiatry complements my current practice like no other specialty could, and has also made me a much better mom, wife, friend, and doctor. A lot of patients come for help with their appearance and end up talking about myriad life issues. For example, if someone sees me for upper-lip laser hair removal, I like to talk about how it feels as a woman to have excessive hair there. Skin care can be so emotional; people cry in my office every day.

I certainly don't let them *leave* crying, but I know it's a positive experience for patients.

When it comes to beauty and a sense of self, these two fields of medicine coalesce brilliantly. So much of how we think affects how we look, and vice versa. I have always believed in treating the body as intrinsically connected to the mind. By virtue of my specialty, I keep up with a lot of other fields of medicine. I refer to ear, nose, and throat doctors all the time, as well as ob-gyns, in vitro specialists, massage therapists, a good spot to get a manicure and pedicure, and even the places to go for the perfect shoes.

Seeking help from a dermatologist should not be viewed as a luxury; it's as important as getting a regular checkup. Like any general practitioner, I see myself as representing the front line of defense for taking better care of yourself so you don't have to resort to radical measures such as plastic surgery, or learn someday that you have a serious form of skin cancer or an age-related disease that threatens your life. Because my techniques aim to lower your stress and heighten your natural beauty, the benefits that await you could be infinite. They will spill over into your heart health, brain health, digestive health, and just about every other aspect of you that makes you, well, *you*.

The reason I left psychiatry to pursue dermatology is simple: I missed the hands-on, physical element of medicine that is so fundamental to dermatology but largely absent from the field of psychiatry. I knew that I was quite adept with my hands and believed I had a calling to use them somehow to take care of more than just people's minds. After all, the essence of being a physician is having the knowledge and opportunity to treat patients' bodies with healing hands and established procedures. I get to do so many different things in dermatology that can truly transform a person's life in a relatively short period of time. Admittedly, there's a definite allure to the immediate gratification that comes with being a dermatologist. A patient can walk into my office and, with one consult or treatment, leave looking and feeling better. That can be difficult to achieve in psychiatry on a regular basis. Skin diseases are interesting, but it's really the interaction with people that is so satisfying.

in this book

Starting in the first chapter, you'll assess your appearance with three separate quizzes, one of which is the groundbreaking SkinAge test that was designed exclusively by RealAge's top scientists to tell you how old your skin is as compared to your chronological age. I'll get you started with revitalizing your looks in chapter 2, and take the confusion out of knowing how to treat your skin daily, weekly, and monthly so it glows naturally. You'll learn the basics of skin care as I go into detail about which beauty products and in-home techniques are worth considering, or are a complete waste of your money. Then, you will prepare to embark on a nine-day journey tailored to your specific needs. Whether you have trouble getting a restful night's sleep, juggling an overbooked schedule, finding time to exercise, or choosing the right foods for your skin, I've got recommendations. You will learn about the seven free habits for healthy skin. These are the habits that support your natural beauty, many of which can encourage cellular restoration. Before you begin the nine-day program, you'll identify which stress profile you match, using a few straightforward questions. This will help you to personalize your program within my day-by-day guidelines outlined in chapter 4, as you learn more fascinating ideas about the intersection of mind and beauty, especially as it relates to your diet, activity level, hormones, age, and lifestyle.

Later in the book, I'll give you an eye-opening peek into your body's dynamic physiology in not only the aging process, but in its response to what you encounter in everyday living. This is when you will begin to fully understand stress aging and the mind-beauty connection. Sprinkled throughout the book you'll find answers to my most frequently asked questions. You will be surprised by how many people come in with the same question but feel like they are the only ones to ask it.

Those who are troubled by particular skin conditions—from acne to skin cancer—will find chapters 8 and 9 especially helpful and encouraging. Then, in the last chapter, I will share all you've ever wanted to know about the more aggressive treatments and procedures available to you should you choose to go that route with a licensed practitioner, and I'll help you find the right doctor, too. This includes straight talk about cosmetic surgery, pharmaceutical interventions, as well as body-image issues that may be weighing too heavily on you. I'll hold nothing back on what I think about certain techniques, some of which are the most popular used today. In all, by the time you're done reading, you'll have accomplished the following steps.

- know your true SkinAge, including how much is physical and how much is emotional
- be ready to complete an easy, practical, and inexpensive nine-day mind-beauty program that can take years—*years*—off your looks
- have found a renewal plan that's right for your psyche, body, and wallet
- have a long-term maintenance regimen that takes only minutes a day and will keep your skin looking and feeling terrific forever

For help in tailoring this program to your body, especially if you have any special health concerns or needs, please speak with your doctor. For example, some of the ideas may not be suitable if you are pregnant and/or breastfeeding. I also encourage you to keep your personal health practitioner in the loop if you plan to commence an exercise program, as suggested in the book, and have not been active in a while. Everyone's response to this program and results will be different. Also be advised that the products and companies mentioned in this book do not reflect an endorsement of any kind, as I currently have no affiliation whatsoever with any of them. I simply want to give you easy, accessible ideas and examples to get you started, because I know so many of you crave specifics and need that extra guidance. I do, however, encourage you to explore other products on the market that may work better for you, or that you may prefer simply for your own reasons. Last, some of the names and identifying characteristics of people described in the book have been changed.

This book is for all of us who have ever looked in the mirror and wished for a better-looking reflection. However, looking in the mirror and seeing a wrinkle you want to eliminate is only part of the equation. Yes, this book keeps a strong focus on skin, but the rewards for making the mind-beauty connection go far beyond a quick fix. I bet many of you will lose unwanted weight, and witness your own medical transformation as you begin to feel healthier and, in a word, alive. Everyone's individual results will be different, but I guarantee that everyone who takes my recommendations and strategies to heart will see and feel an improvement, however big or small, on both the inside and outside. We all deserve to look and feel our best, no matter how young or old the calendar says we are. Ready for a whole new you? Turn the page and let's get going!

Bonus: Go to www.RealAge.com for additional support, resources, and information that will optimize your program.

the mind-beauty connection

1

the skinage test and other reality checks

*How Do You **Really** Feel About Your Looks?*

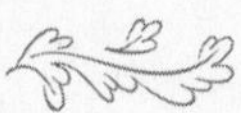

Admit it: At some time or another (perhaps many times), you looked in the mirror and thought, "Where did *that* come from?" I wish I had a dime for every time a woman said this to herself; I'd be the richest person on earth. I think the experience is shared among all of us, and, when this question first crosses your mind, it gets you to examine more than just one particular spot. Suddenly, you feel the need to take a closer look all over. So you then follow the tracks of previously unrecognized wrinkles across your forehead, a discolored area or brown spot on your cheeks, and the genesis of a deeply rooted pimple on your chin. You step back to take inventory of other body parts. Hair. Neck. Chest (*décolletage*). Hands. Hips. Waistline. Profile. You don't look like you did ten, maybe even just two, years ago. An ugly, sinking feeling washes over you. Your face—correction, your whole body—is morphing and you can't control it. Or at least you *think* you can't control it. Yes, you are getting older and can no longer be mistaken for a youth (the days of getting carded to buy alcohol are over). I bet you wouldn't want to be a kid again anyhow, but still, you wouldn't mind having the energy and vibrant looks of one.

Here's the good news: You can do something to rejuvenate the appearance that the stress of modern life has stolen. That's right: A lot of what you see is *reversible*. And the program described in this book will also help you recapture the energy and vitality that life has momentarily confiscated.

Who knew that a little word like *aging* could conjure so much emotion. None of us really thinks about it until we see evidence of it in the mirror one random day.

The Age-Old Question

When does aging start? Well, at some point during your adolescence—between about eleven and twenty-five years old—the accelerated rate of cellular growth in your body began to slow down. In other words, you began to age. And while you may not have noticed this change on the outside or felt anything downshift on the inside, it marked the beginning of the slow, inevitable decline we all experience as the years go by.

It doesn't take a doctor like me to tell you that, over time, the first signs of aging become evident and the skin, which is our largest organ, accounting for 12 to 16 percent of the body weight, reveals the first clues of this process. This is when we notice wrinkling, creasing, dryness, and drooping . . . and perhaps have that sad moment in front of a mirror. While it may seem to come on suddenly (*my face changed overnight!*), it has, in fact, been slowly coming about day after day, year after year. You probably knew that, too. No one etched your face in the middle of the night because you had a bad day or week. Don't blame your spouse, your kids, your job, your financial troubles, or weight woes, and don't you dare blame yourself. We've all had those moments; they are uniquely human. Luckily, we don't have to resign ourselves to the thought there is nothing we can do about it.

The cyclical process of *cellular turnover*—the complex phenomenon of tissue growth, repair, and breakdown—says a lot about how we age. When we think of aging on the outside, we are really talking about how fast our collagen and elastin, which are the protein fibers that keep our skin springy, resilient, and vibrant, deteriorate. Once damaged, these fibers become dry and brittle, leading to wrinkles and sagging.

When does this collision course for collagen really pick up pace? Most people start to complain around the age of thirty-five. That is when the breakdown speeds up; and keeping the twentysomething appearance (with taut, dewy, and fresh skin worthy of a magazine cover) gets to be an uphill battle. On the bright side, your lifestyle plays a lead role in your health and looks. And no matter what cards you think your mom and dad dealt you when you were born, you can hold the remote control to your appearance and come out looking beautiful. Top health institutions now agree that 70 to 80 percent of our health and longevity is up to us. In other words, the decisions we make and habits we keep account for at least 70 percent of our health (and, in that regard, our appearance). Now, that's an empowering fact. So, the time has come to live the most beautiful life with the best strategies to looking and feeling terrific.

By the time you finish this book, you'll be on your way to looking younger and fresher, and having skin that's healthier and happier than it's been in a long time. And ironically, the more tired and stressed you are, the bigger the difference you'll see. Along the way you are going to learn a lot about the aging process in general. We can't talk about skin and beauty without a discussion about aging and health in general for that matter. These are all interconnected; the actions you take to repair and rejuvenate the outside will also give your interiors a much-needed improvement.

An Age-Old Pursuit

All civilizations have looked for the fountain of youth and attempted to reverse the signs and effects of aging. The bonus for living in the twenty-first century: We know more than ever now about the aging process and how not only to address it, but also to physically *reverse* it. You will be delightfully surprised by some of my recommendations, which can remove years from you without breaking the bank.

Just as our skin cells need a constant supply of water, oxygen, vitamins, and nutrients, so does every organ and tissue in our body, from our brain and heart down to the tendons in our toes. And, just as we will be revitalizing the connective tissues in our skin, we also will be addressing similar connective tissues on the inside—in blood vessels, nerves, joints, tendons, and ligaments. The state of all these body parts has a profound say in how well we age, how beautiful we look, and how long we live. Tackling inflammation on the outside, including conditions like acne, eczema, rosacea, and so on, can result in treating inflammation on the inside, too. Inflammation, by the way, will be a topic of discussion throughout this book, because it's at the core of *ugliness*. I say that in reference to what we don't like to see when we look at ourselves in the mirror, as well as what we don't want to hear from our doctors in the exam room.

Remember!

Don't forget to go to my center at www.RealAge.com for supplemental support, updates, and online access to resources that will further assist you in this program. You can also take the following tests on the site, too.

As stated in the introduction, this book aims to enhance everything about you—mind, body, and quality of life. The goal, of course, that we all want to achieve is to shorten the time we spend sick or diseased—in other words (and to echo the late anthropologist Ashley Montagu), to die as youthful as we can but as *late* as we can.

The very first step in this journey, however, is understanding two things: how you really feel about your looks and what you can do to see a better, more vibrant you tomorrow. The next chapter deals with number two. For now, let's focus on where you currently stand by taking three tests. Consider this the starting point from which you can set goals and begin to track successes as you move forward and welcome all the benefits that can await you in this beauty program. The time has come to celebrate the demise of wrinkles, age spots, puffy eyes, chronic exhaustion, and so much more.

test 1: the quickie

This test takes all of five seconds. It's a simple gut check to assess how you feel about your skin this moment. While it's certainly okay to focus on your facial skin, I recommend thinking about your skin all over your body. After all, looks go much further than the face; if that mole on your belly or those spider veins on your legs really bother you, you'll think about them immediately. Don't look in the mirror. Don't think about it for more than a few seconds. Just check which face below expresses how you feel about how you currently look.

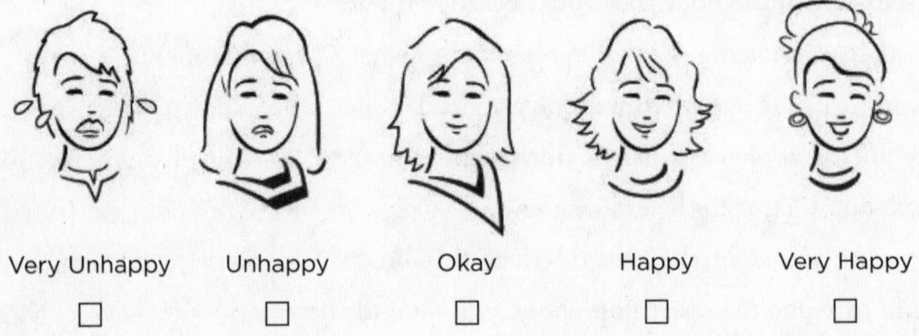

While this test may be simple, it reveals the type of journey you'll take in this book. If you selected "Happy" or "Very Happy," you're more content with your appearance than most. But if you answered anything from "Okay" to "Very Unhappy," I suspect you have the same internal conversation going on that a lot of my patients do. It's often a running commentary, and it's likely to be loudest and most insistent when you're looking in a magnifying mirror. It goes like this:

- I have bad skin. No, I have good skin. No, my skin used to be good and now it's bad.
- Where did this wrinkle come from? Did I get it overnight? Omigod, I'm getting old!
- All of a sudden I have to wear all this makeup. I never had to before. What's happening here?

- I've got acne? I haven't had zits since my twenties! Where did these pimples come from?

- If I see these bags under my eyes one more day, I'll scream! Okay, so I only got four hours of sleep last night, but when am I ever going to make up for all the sleep I've lost?

Sound familiar? These are just the short versions. Sometimes the stream-of-skin-consciousness in your head plays endlessly, going on and on in a maddening loop. Are you ready to hit the stop button once and for all? Then let's put some real science to work with the second test: finding out your true SkinAge.

This is not an ordinary beauty quiz, the kind that make brief, monthly appearances in most fashion magazines and then vanish forever. Two of the scientists who devised the RealAge test, which involved reviewing more than 30,000 studies to find the 100-plus factors that determine your body's biological age, developed the SkinAge test. Alex Goetz, MD, PhD, and Harriet Imrey, PhD, dug into the research, went through a decade's worth of scholarly papers, compared countless causes and key effects of skin aging, then boiled down the data to find a scientifically valid way to measure SkinAge—that is, to give you a real fix on how old you *look* versus how old you *are*.

What they came up with is brilliant in its simplicity: Instead of assessing your exposure to the endless variables that can cause skin aging—genes, sun habits, whether you ever smoked, stress levels, ethnic background, if you have an indoor or outside job, where you live, pollution factors, and so on—they looked only at the results: how many signs of aging actually exist on your face. The test here entails just thirteen questions, but it's a very reliable SkinAge predictor. For those interested in taking this to a deeper level, you can use an even more precise calculator at www.RealAge.com. As a bonus, the site will do the scoring for you.

For the SkinAge test to work, you must be between the ages of 27 and 81. Why the cut-off points? If you're younger than twenty-seven, you don't have enough visible aging yet to measure. If you're older than eighty-one, the gap between your SkinAge and your calendar age won't be significant.

Ready? It's time to find out if your SkinAge is younger, older, or the same as your body age. (Oh, and if you also want to find out your entire body's RealAge—how old you are biologically, not according to the calendar—you can take the free test at the RealAge site.)

the skinage test

Sometimes we don't see ourselves very clearly. Take this test right after you've washed your face or gotten out of the shower. Dry off, rub in some moisturizer (it won't affect your visual exam), then take a good look in the mirror as you answer these questions. Add up your score using the box below to find out your SkinAge. Try not to cheat! If any of these questions brings you to see something you didn't notice before, or that you wish to avoid acknowledging, 'fess up! This is your chance to take inventory of your looks—face them dead on and be honest. Only then can you effectively take action to turn back the clock. Also avoid pulling or tugging on your skin as you do this to influence your answers. No one is watching you and you won't be graded, so be true to yourself.

1. *Is the skin of your cheeks (and maybe your forehead, too) smooth or sagging?*

a) Smooth
b) Somewhat sagging
c) Sagging and forming jowls on my jawline

2. *Do you have bags under your eyes?*

a) No
b) Small ones
c) Distinct bags

3. *Are your upper eyelids drooping, almost touching your upper lashes?*

a) No
b) Slightly
c) Definitely

4. *Do you see fine lines on your forehead and/or cheeks?*

a) No
b) Some
c) Quite a few

5. *Do you see deep wrinkles on your cheeks?*

a) No
b) Yes, some deepening wrinkles
c) Yes, several deep wrinkles

6. *Do you see smile lines leading from the corners of your nostrils to the corners of your mouth?*

a) No
b) Yes, soft lines
c) Yes, very clear lines

7. *Do you see crow's feet at the outer corners of your eyes?*

a) No
b) Yes, slight lines
c) Yes, marked lines

8. *Do you see wrinkles under your eyes?*

a) No
b) Yes, fine wrinkles
c) Yes, very marked wrinkles

9. *Are there any frown lines running horizontally across your forehead and/ or vertically between your eyebrows?*

a) No
b) Yes, slight lines
c) Yes, very marked lines

10. *Do you see fine vertical lines above your upper lip?*

a) No
b) Yes, a few
c) Yes, many

11. *Do you see fine up-and-down lines on your lips?*

a) No
b) Yes, some
c) Yes, many

12. *Instead of the coloring on your cheeks or forehead being even, do you have any small red dots or uneven coloring?*

a) No
b) Some dots or uneven coloring
c) A lot of dots and uneven coloring

13. *Do you have any milia on your forehead or cheeks (**milia** are small bumps that look like little whiteheads but don't go away)?*

a) No
b) Yes

Determining Your SkinAge

Now we're ready to figure out just how young or old your skin really is. Circle the points for each answer, then add them up.

1. a=0
   b=3
   c=6
2. a=0
   b=1.5
   c=3
3. a=0
   b=1.5
   c=3
4. a=0
   b=1.5
   c=2.5
5. a=0
   b=1
   c=2
6. a=0
   b=0.5
   c=1.5
7. a=0
   b=0.5
   c=1.5
8. a=0
   b=0.5
   c=1.5
9. a=0
   b=0.5
   c=1.5
10. a=0
    b=1
    c=2
11. a=0
    b=1
    c=2
12. a=0
    b=7
    c=14
13. a=0
    b=5

Total points ____ + 27 = ____ Your SkinAge!

Is your SkinAge younger, the same, or older than your chronological age? If it's more, don't panic. Just imagine how good you're going to feel when you can take six years or more off your SkinAge. That, and you living the rest of your life with the healthiest, best-looking skin you can have, is my goal.

the self-image test

This final test determines what your body language reveals about *you*. How you look on the outside and what is actually happening inside at the cellular level, especially in the brain, given your emotions, mood, and overall stress level, go hand in hand. You cannot spot treat your body without taking in and evaluating your whole being.

Whenever someone comes into my office—male or female, for the first time or the tenth—the psych part of my brain automatically springs into action. While we're meeting and greeting, I instinctively speed-read their body language, checking for signs of emotional stress that might be involved in whatever skin problems triggered the appointment. If there seem to be more than skin-deep issues at play, I need to address those too when I'm figuring out what treatments to prescribe.

These are the nine questions that go through my mind when I see any patient. Ask them about yourself, jotting down your answers either right in this book, on a piece of paper, or in a journal if you keep one. This won't take long, but be thoughtful and frank; don't cheat by predicting what you think would be a good or correct answer. The more honest you are about yourself, the better you can achieve the results you want with the knowledge you gain in the book. It's okay if some of these questions get you thinking, but try to avoid overanalyzing these particular questions, or which answers are the right ones. Simply think about how you normally look when you go out, and not necessarily how you look while you're curled up with this book. After you take the test, I'll show you how to decode your body language the way I would if we were meeting in my office for a personal consultation.

1. *How do you wear your hair?*

2. *Do you pluck or wax your eyebrows?*

3. *Does your mom (sister, best friend) still nag at you to stand up straight?*

4. *When it comes to makeup, do you normally wear:*

   [ ] little or none   [ ] a moderate amount   [ ] the works

5. *Are your hands more likely to be touching your face or in your lap?*

6. *Do you usually wear fitted clothes or loose ones?*

7. *Describe your normal walk. Is it more:*

   [ ] slow and ambling   [ ] quick and intent

8. *When you talk to people, do you tend to look directly at them or let your eyes roam around the room?*

9. *Do you try to quickly check your appearance before meeting people?*

What Your Body Language Is Telling You

Here's what I'm looking for when I scan someone's appearance. See how this compares with your answers to get a clear idea of the signals you're silently telegraphing to the world—and to yourself, if you're listening. (Some of these may sound like generalizations, but they do happen to reflect clinical evidence that I—and most other doctors—have witnessed in practice. There are some gray areas here, and not every interpretation is black-and-white, but I encourage you to be as open as you can to the following explanations and see if you can pinpoint where you are on the spectrum of possibilities.)

- Extralong bangs or sideswept hair that half covers your face can be a dramatic style statement, but sometimes suggests that you're covering up something (acne, aging?) or a little nervous around people.

Regardless of what hairstyles are in or out at the moment, a woman who is self-confident tends to wear her hair in a way that reveals her face and accentuates her features. Whether it's pulled back, piled up, or tucked behind an ear, it broadcasts: *I feel good about how I look.* Women who are self-conscious about themselves or worried about their skin often use their hair as a barrier or cover-up, or disguise.

- *Untouched or heavily plucked eyebrows both get my attention.*

When I see a woman who has thick, heavy brows with stray hairs across the top of her nose, self-esteem questions register with me, particularly if she has also made little effort with her hair or makeup. It implies that spending time on herself doesn't seem worth the effort. At the other extreme, over-plucked brows suggests a tendency toward obsessiveness that could also involve picking at the skin, something dermatologists always worry about (see "If you constantly touch your face").

- *When you sit, do you slump? When you stand, do you hunch?*

Either one can signal a few things: exhaustion, self-consciousness, poor muscle tone, some depression, or just a woman who is not quite comfortable with her height. That happened to me as a kid: I grew fast and early, outstripping half my class, and started slumping to fit in better physically. My mom helped me understand the good things about being tall (i.e., playing sports, reaching top shelves, and raiding her closet) and now I wish I were even taller than my five feet, eight inches. As a result, I'm really tuned in to people who don't stand up straight. Is it because they are too tired . . . or down in the dumps? Ironically, that's when good posture is more important than ever, because slumping makes it harder to breathe deeply and the resulting lack of oxygen can make you feel even gloomier, not to mention tired.

The Power of a Profile, or How to Look Taller, Thinner, Younger, and More Confident in Fewer than Ten Seconds: Stand up straight! Posture, which is essentially how we hold ourselves up and position our bodies whether sitting or standing, plays a big part in how we look and feel. It can also help us to stay stronger and flexible as we get older. I think everyone can improve on this. Imagine someone pulling a string up through your body, from your feet up through your head. Everything gets lined up and there is no part having to resist gravity. When sitting, see if you can pull your chest up (avoid slouching forward or leaning back), shoulders down (not up by your ears) and relaxed with your head lined up right over them. If you're in front of a computer screen, make sure it's level with your eyes. Uncross your knees or feet and bend them at a ninety-degree angle. Here's a challenge: See if you can go a day without cradling a cell phone in between your ears and shoulders; switch which shoulder carries the purse, and rely on the hand that doesn't normally carry items to lift and tote. Taking up yoga or Pilates can also help you to focus on how you carry yourself; these practices are all about finding body balance and strengthening the muscles that will naturally allow you to maintain an elegant, slimming profile.

- *The messages that your makeup can send.*

It can be a tip-off to everything from where you were born to how full your calendar is. No makeup is often a statement. It's up to me—and, in this case, you—to figure out what it's saying. That you prefer to be all natural? That you don't feel very feminine? Or that you're too busy to even swipe on some lipstick? It can be hard to judge someone who prefers to wear no makeup, because people can have uniquely different reasons for avoiding makeup. Because makeup is so much a part of our culture I question whether the person is having problems with self-confidence and self-esteem to the point where she doesn't have the motivation to use any.

When we are sick, sad, tired, or just relaxing over the weekend we typically forgo the makeup. It's rare to meet someone so overly confident that she vows to show off her natural looks by going bare on a regular basis (hey, even supermodels usually wear makeup when in public). The right amount of makeup can do wonders for our self-perception, which then relates directly with self-confidence. If you don't like to wear makeup because you fear it's the root of your skin troubles, you will love my ideas in chapter 3. News flash: Bad skin does not have to be related to makeup. In fact, rarely do skin issues arise from reactions with makeup or products. They arise from mistreating your skin.

Light to moderate makeup is pretty straightforward. It says that you don't have much to hide—acne scars, discolorations, undereye circles. Unless it seems more haphazard than deliberate, chances are you're basically comfortable with your looks.

Heavy makeup almost always makes me wonder if someone's covering up something, from breakouts to a birthmark. But—big exception here—sometimes wearing quite a bit of makeup is traditional: It's practically a birthright in much of the South and in Texas. On the other hand, some women use makeup as a social mask. When they say, "I can't go out without my face on," they mean it. They want the world to see them in one unchanging, perfect way—even though nothing's ever perfect and life changes constantly.

- *If you constantly touch your face, think about why you do.*

Some people are trying to hide crooked teeth. Others may be uncomfortable about showing their emotions. But what I'm really looking for here are what skin doctors call pickers. I mentally divide patients into pickers and nonpickers. If a nonpicker has a mosquito bite, she tries not to scratch it; if she has a scab, she generally leaves it alone. Pickers, on the other hand, are often anxious and can't leave anything alone—flaky areas, skin tags, small sores, ragged cuticles, peeling sunburns, they'll go at them all relentlessly. And picking always, always gets worse with stress.

What's the big deal? Persistent picking discolors and scars. I'm forever telling patients to stop touching their faces because the first step is to become conscious that they're doing it—not everyone is aware of it. Next, I ask pickers if they use a magnifying mirror and tell them to throw it away if they do. Examining their skin in minute detail seems to feed the urge to pick. Of course, picking can just be a reaction to stress ("When I'm tense, I pick, twist my hair, chew my nails") but if it turns into a habit, it's a hard one to break. That's why I always try to nip it in the bud.

Being a picker may be hardwired a little bit, or modeled after a parent. Some people are wrongly taught to, say, pop pimples. I see kids pick and prod at themselves when they are anxious, and this continues into adulthood although it may take other forms. Most people who pick are aware that they do it, but in the moment it can be a mindless act, which is why trying to be more mindful of what triggers the picking, and finding methods to break the habit through healthy alternatives to the act, is important.

Most pickers do it at the end of the day in the comfort of home. This is when they are no longer distracted by work, plus they know it's not socially acceptable to pick in public. But, in the evening, our underlying worries grow bigger as the day slows down. Now we have time to mull over our woes and for some, picking at scars, scabs, or acne is relieving. I once had a patient who broke down to me about how she and her husband bought a vacation house on the beach in an isolated area. Her husband worked out of town a lot, so she would retreat to their second home while he was away on business. While she was there, in her loneliness (the trigger) she would start picking and manipulating her face with tweezers in the magnifying mirror they had in the bathroom. She said she never picked when her husband was home, but was troubled by her behavior when left alone in this particular bathroom with a gigantic mirror.

Our first order of business was alerting her husband to the problem. She brought him into my office and I explained how he could help her avoid the constant picking that was doing a number on her face. Throwing out the mirror was also on the agenda. When people don't have a partner they can rely upon to help them in this manner, I recommend that patients gain a better awareness of their picking so when they feel the urge to pick, they can switch gears by calling a friend or reading a book. If picking happens as a result of a sore or itch, an ice pack or cold compresses can be very helpful. A little hydrocortisone cream on an incessant itch or a milk bath will also squelch the flames, and the urge to touch it.

- *If most of your clothes are fitted or baggy, that can be a clue too.*

Sure, this is a generalization, but the more comfortable you are with yourself and your body, the more likely you are to wear clothes that set off its shape. For instance, if someone comes in with a thin face who is wearing lots and lots of layers, I wonder if she is hiding anorexia. If someone comes in with a full face who is wearing lots of layers, I wonder about recent weight gain. But if someone comes in who is a little heavy but wearing well-fitted clothes, I suspect that she's lost some weight and is proud of it. If a normal-weight woman arrives in baggy clothes, though, it might suggest the reverse. If all four look like they dressed carefully, it suggests—whew—a sense of self-worth. All of us use clothing to say things about ourselves; think about what your message usually is.

- *How you walk is a major confidence clue.*

When you cover ground with energy and motivation, it telegraphs to the world that you are self-assured, in charge of yourself, and full of life. When you don't, the message is just the opposite. Slow, shuffling walks don't just say you're vulnerable, they shout it: Women who become the targets of street crime have been proven in studies to walk with slower, less purposeful, less confident strides.

- *Social ease is often seen in the eyes.*

Avoiding eye contact suggests anxiety, depression, embarrassment, shyness, or just vague discomfort. Sometimes, of course, people are just nervous about being around a doctor. Or they may have this distorted sense that they have done something bad, such as let themselves go physically, and that I am going to lecture them about it. Maybe they're uneasy about why they came in—"It's only a little rash but, you know, it's down there." Maybe they think I'll judge them for wanting Botox. Maybe they feel silly—"It's just a few pimples." To make them feel more comfortable, I share personal stories (about my horrendous high school acne) or show them where I use Botox myself (a little between my brows). But if someone constantly avoids eye contact, even after a few appointments, when we seem to have established a good relationship, I'll bring it up and say, "I notice you have a hard time looking at me. Do you know that you're doing that? Does it ever happen at work or on a date? Do you realize that it makes you seem nervous or shy?" It's something I keep working on. I want to see it improve over time.

- *If you don't check your appearance before meeting people, why not?*

Before seeing any patient, I take a quick look in a mirror and check my teeth (especially right after lunch!), maybe put on a bit of lipstick or smooth my hair. This isn't just trying to present myself well. It also shows my respect for the people who've made the trip to see me, whether they came from two streets or two states away.

If you don't make a little spruce-up effort when you're about to see someone, is it because you don't think it will make a difference . . . or you really don't care how you look . . . or you just never have time to give yourself a second glance? All three bring up questions. If you're always putting your kids before yourself, or you're insanely overscheduled, or you think your looks are beyond help . . . you're neglecting and/or undervaluing yourself. It's time to give yourself permission to take care of you!

congrats

The hard part is over. Self-examination can be tough, but hopefully these tests have helped you to understand where you are on the SkinAge test and how your physical appearance ties into your emotions and sense of self. You'll be getting a full dose of information coming up in later chapters that will help you to truly see the connection between your mind and body. The science is stunning. And I think that the more information you have, the less fear you'll have about aging.

My goal in this chapter was simply to help you take a first look at the physical and psychological factors contributing to your skin's looks and health. Now let's fast-forward and get right to those recommendations that will turn back the clock and help you to reverse the signs of aging. You'll be able to set your personalized program in motion today.

2

getting started with revitalizing your looks

Skin-Care Essentials

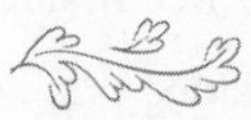

Meet Clarissa, a thirty-five-year-old mother with a skin age of at least thirty-nine. On some days, it's more like forty-two. Like so many other working moms trying to have—and do—it all, Clarissa doesn't get enough sleep at night (between five and six hours). The product manager for a large company in San Diego sets her alarm for 6:15 every morning so she can get her two young twins dressed and fed before dropping them off at preschool on her way to work. She's at her desk by 9:00 A.M. to do a job that has become even more demanding due to a recent promotion. She's usually back home around 7:00 P.M. Her husband—whose workday starts and ends much earlier than hers—is the family chef. He's fed the twins by the time Clarissa walks in, and while he pulls together some food for her, Clarissa does bath time with the kids. After that, the parents usually grab a half hour together while the kids wind down. They head to bed around nine and Dad's close behind them, as he's up at four. After they'e gone to bed Clarissa starts the Internet part of her night, catching up with friends via e-mail, checking the news, surfing her fave sites, and often doing some work. It pushes her bedtime into the wee hours.

The sleep deficit, caused in part by her stimulating, late-night Internet addiction as she catches up with friends on e-mail and surfs the net, has begun to show up on her face in the form of crinkles and a dullish skin tone, making her look older than her thirty-five years. "No one calls me, even by mistake, 'young lady' anymore," she says, laughing. She also has dry white patches on her cheeks, a few horizontal lines on her forehead, and some sun spots that, she emphasizes, are *not* from the recent past. "Whenever I go for a half-hour run, I always wear a hat to cover my face and big sunglasses. Living in San Diego, I see a lot of sun damage, and I'm terrified of it." To prove it, she brandishes a bottle of Shiseido sunscreen with an SPF of fifty-five. "I love this and use it every morning, rain or shine," she says.

I gave Clarissa a big thumbs-up to this healthy habit during her first appointment. Like most of my patients, she asked for a low-maintenance skin regimen, explaining, "I barely have time to brush my hair in the morning." After taking her history (no blistering sunburns as a child but some secondhand smoke from her dad), I decided that topical *tretinoin* (under the trade name Renova .02) would be an easy fix for Clarissa's fine lines, wrinkles, and brown spots, if she used it regularly every night. To treat the dry white patches, I gave her a product sample of hydrocortisone, which cleared them immediately.

Filling a prescription for Renova was the easiest of the antiaging tasks. I wanted Clarissa to go much further in addressing underlying stress. Clarissa's life had become a treadmill of working and taking care of the kids, and I knew that from being a mom myself, having three-year-old twins wasn't easy. I encouraged her to sleep more, and take more time-outs without the kids so she could focus more on the happiness factor with her husband. I recommended that she hire a babysitter and go out at least every other weekend.

Six months later, Clarissa reported great results. Her skin, and her lifestyle, had improved measurably. Her skin tone evened out, and her sun spots faded. "My skin feels firmer, and the texture is so smooth that it looks like I'm wearing powder, though I'm not. I haven't needed it since about a month or so after I started on the Renova." She did have a few trouble spots—dry areas around her chin and jawline—but I instructed her to avoid applying the Renova to that area for about a week and it worked brilliantly.

Through trial and error, Clarissa also found a doable nightly skin routine she likes and has down pat: washing her face during her evening shower with her favorite Kiehl's cleanser, then applying Renova, and last a hydrating moisturizer from Lancôme. (Mornings involve just a quick cleanse and a slathering of Shiseido sunscreen.) The evening self-care adds a bit of constancy to her busy life, a bit of me time that she finds therapeutic. "By being more diligent about my skin-care regimen, I feel proactive, like I'm actually helping improve the health of my skin. And knowing that I'm making my skin look and act younger makes me feel better."

Getting more help has been good, too. Clarissa's sister-in-law babysits for the couple two weekends a month so they can have some quality time together. This self-described workaholic known to bring her job home has also managed to shave a few hours off her workweek. While she is trying to go to bed earlier—for her, that means eleven—Clarissa admits to falling off the wagon at times. "I'm probably averaging about six and one-half to seven hours of sleep a night, which is more than I used to get," she says. "But sometimes I toss and turn. Some people can just go to sleep when their head hits the pillow—my husband, for one; he's lucky that way, but not me. My mind starts to race."

Clarissa is not alone with her sleep issues. The same tips I gave her for achieving better, more restful sleep at night I'll be giving you a bit later. One fact that Clarissa's story points out is that skin care doesn't have to be an expensive, time-consuming proposition. Whatever your age, and no matter how many kids or daily dramas you juggle, you can look younger—now *and* later—if you adopt a few stress-busters that really work for you, know which skin products actually do something (and which aren't worth a dime), develop healthy sun habits, and learn how to deal with adult acne if that's a problem for you. Sure, starting early and being consistent are ideal but . . . it's never too late to trade so-so habits for super ones.

Many women overdo it with their skin: overclean, overtreat, overeverything. So we're going to go all the way back to basics during this program. Give your skin a rest by doing the absolute minimum. Imagine doing less, but seeing greater results.

In this chapter I'm going to cover beauty basics—what I think every woman should do regularly no matter what kind of skin she has. I'll also share my own personal everyday skin-care routine, which can set the foundation for your new skin-care regimen. To start, let's explore some of the general products currently available on the market—virtually all of them touting something related to youth, beauty, and antiaging. I'm going to show you how to save yourself money, headaches, wrinkles, and regrets.

The Must-Haves for Optimum Skin Beauty

- A gentle daily cleanser
- Two good moisturizers—one for day use with sunscreen (SPF 30+) and another for night use
- If necessary: antiacne washes and formulas, exfoliants, antioxidant serums, retinoid/retinol formulas.

FYI: Several skin-care companies have approached me to do a collaborative line of products, but I've turned them all down so far. Unless I love something and really believe it works, I'd never put my name on it. You'll find plenty of brand-name ideas in this book, but don't let my ideas stop you from experimenting with others. The key is to find what works for you personally.

antiaging products: what really works

In 2005, American women dropped a cool $664 million on antiaging creams and potions, and that was just in department stores. Today, that figure has jumped to nearly $2 *billion*. We're shelling out big bucks for ingredients like oil from the seeds of hand-harvested arctic cranberries and Koishimaru silk extracted from delicate cocoons. And if you add cosmetics in general that we buy to spruce up our natural looks (or cover up those blemishes and uneven skin tones) then the number skyrockets well into the billions.

Maddeningly, much of that money is being spent on products that have little effect on skin's aging process, because to halt the march of fine lines, sag, and pigmentation changes, you have to change skin's deeper layers. And if any of the bazillion department and drugstore products that claim to erase age's treadmarks could actually *do* that—say, by increasing cell turnover in the dermis—the FDA would classify them as drugs. A few do exist, but you can only buy them with a doctor's prescription (see the section on retinoids).

Why are so many cosmetic claims so convincing? Five reasons:

Expensive Vocab

A cosmeceutical is any over-the-counter skin treatment that is not considered a cosmetic or pharmaceutical, but a largely unregulated hybrid of the two. Put another way, it's a cosmetic product *claiming* to have medicinal or druglike benefits. In 2006, it was estimated that that U.S. sales of skin-care cosmeceuticals had reached $6.4 billion annually, and those sales continue to grow.

- **Clever writing.** Read the claims carefully and you'll realize they're full of qualifying words like "aim to" and "designed to diminish" and "reduce the appearance of" and . . . well, you get the idea. These promises are etched in anything but stone.

- **Scientific trappings.** Even if a product says, "clinically shown to . . ." remember that it's one thing to research how a component of coffee, such as caffeine, say, affects mouse skin, and quite another to claim that adding coffee to a lotion will perk up human skin. Also, little cosmetic research meets the scientific gold standard—that is, a randomized, double-blind crossover study, performed by a qualified researcher (who is usually affiliated with a university or teaching hospital) with no financial stake in the outcome. The studies are usually very small, typically lack a control for comparison, and are paid for by cosmetics companies, which have a vested interest in the results.

- **The placebo effect.** If you've just plunked down $27.50, or $275, for a moisturizer, you want it to make your skin look younger, smoother, firmer, so it's easy to see changes for the better. And let's not forget the psychological aspect of buying something luxuriously packaged. The packaging alone can lead to you believe it will work! Savvy beauty companies don't skimp on presentation, especially when they command mucho dinero for their goods.
- **No cops.** Cosmetics aren't regulated by the FDA, so if a product doesn't diminish fine lines, well, nothing really happens. And if you're not sure it did anything unusual, but it smelled wonderful and felt terrific, you might buy it again anyway.
- **Vague promises.** How many times have you seen a product marketed with the phrase "Clinically proven to reduce the appearance of fine lines and wrinkles by up to 33 percent," or some such? Have you ever asked yourself, What does that mean, exactly? You don't live in a clinical setting, so does that percentage work in the real world? The term *clinically proven* sounds persuasive, but as we just saw under "scientific trappings," it's often more marketing than science. Generally, the phrase means that at least one component of the product has been shown, in one study or another, to have had some biological action, such as helping wounds heal faster by stimulating cell division. But it's not necessarily true that it has been demonstrated by a well-controlled, independent clinical study to have significant effects in skin.

Paying for Pearls, But Seeing the Same Old Skin

When *Forbes* magazine reviewed the world's most expensive age-defying facial products, they found that the average price of the top ten products on their list cost $402 *per ounce*. That's 7,500 percent more than the price of products sold at most drug and grocery stores. What makes these products so expensive? Other than hype and heavy marketing (that you pay for!), many include exotic (read: *expensive*) ingredients like caviar, crushed pearls, and extracts from rare plants from remote terrain. Antioxidants like grape-seed extract, chamomile oils, and alpha lipoic acid—all of which are touted to fight the free radicals that ravage skin tissue—also drive up the price. Add to that the customized cell messenger proteins, which allegedly stimulate cell growth and which I think are bogus, and you've got yourself a spendy package.

That said, earlier this year scientists put a price on happiness. You know what I mean—how much we enjoy paying for something really really expensive once in a while. I personally think it goes a little deeper than retail therapy. Who doesn't get a tad more satisfaction from designer brands, be it a purse or a lotion, than from cheaper versions, even if they are exactly the same? Sounds ridiculous, but I think every woman can agree. And now, it has been proven: The more we believe an item is worth, the happier we are with our purchase (at least for a short time). In a study that I wish I had participated in because it sounds like so much fun, participants were hooked up to brain-scan machines and told to take a sip from five glasses of wine, which ranged from five dollars to ninety dollars per bottle. When they were told they were drinking a glass of wine from a ninety-dollar bottle, brain scans showed increased activity in the medial orbital frontal cortex, the area of the brain that registers pleasure. The hilarious part is that these people's pleasure spots activated in the brain even when they were fooled to think they were drinking a ninety-dollar bottle when, in fact, they were swilling cheap vino that retails for around five dollars!

It's practically instinctual to believe that when you pay more, you get more—that a higher price commands a higher quality. The kicker here is that

Q: Do expensive skin-care products work better than drugstore brands?

A: Not often! Many drugstore brands are excellent, and the larger companies spend a lot of money on research and development of their products. Expensive products sometimes feel better when they are applied, because those companies spend more money on the vehicles that the products are in. Buying an expensive product feels special to some people, and that's okay as long as the products do not irritate or make your skin break out. For me, I get to try many products, drugstore and expensive, and I use many drugstore brands that are both hypoallergenic and fragrance free, as I have very sensitive skin. There are some expensive sunscreens from France that I think are worth every penny.

Q: What do you think of the increasingly popular organic beauty lines—you know, the ones whose ingredient lists read almost like food labels?

A: I get asked this a lot because they are extremely trendy, especially now that we're all trying to be more green in the way we live. The intentions of these companies are great but I have one big concern: Almost all of them use many, many plant extracts, from apples and mint to cactus and soy. However, a lot of plants can be irritating. Think of poison ivy, for heaven's sake; it's completely natural and organic! Sure, it's an extreme example, but even aloe, which everyone thinks of as the ultimate soother, is an irritant for some people. So is lavender: It upsets some people's skin more than itchy wool clothing. Also, if you read the ingredients labels on many so-called natural products, they are at least as long as those on some mainstream products, yet there is often very little research on many of the ingredients. Bottom line: I'm cautious with these.

---

if you *believe* something better is happening to you (like you're getting to drink fine wine, or, in the case of cosmetics, indulge yourself with uberluxurious product lines sworn by by the celebrities in haute-couture fashion magazines), you essentially affect the way your brain handles the experience. By the way, the researchers in this latest study discovered that this effect happens across all types of purchases, and is not isolated to wine-tasting circles. Granted, some people can confuse an item's worth with their own self-worth (as in, "Will *this* make me happy?"), but that's another can of worms. Suffice it to say that I give you permission to splurge when you feel it's appropriate . . . and really want to. The occasional splurge can knock your stress down a notch or two. Just don't start thinking that happiness is only a purchase away. You know the old cliché: You can't buy happiness.

The Only Proven Wrinkle Reducers and Age Fighters: Retinoids

Thankfully, they do exist. There aren't many of them, but they work. Two are prescription-only derivatives of vitamin A: *tretinoin* (brand names: Retin-A, Avita, Renova, which is the product I prescribed for Clarissa, and others) and *tazarotene* (Tazorac, Avage). Called retinoids, these are FDA-approved, rub-on treatments that rank high on my list of skin-renewal candidates. I regularly prescribe them in my practice, and they can be applied to the neck, chest, hands, and forearms in addition to the face. You would start by applying the treatment twice weekly—at night while your skin is naturally recuperating. This helps you minimize the irritation that usually accompanies the treatment when you first start out. Then, you would increase how often you use it, with the goal of applying it every night.

It takes several weeks to start seeing results, but prescription retinoids can transform your skin, smoothing wrinkles, unclogging pores, lightening superficial brown spots, and improving the texture of the skin. They go to town on acne, and can be used to treat other skin conditions, such as psoriasis, all of which we'll discuss later. Retinoids can actually regenerate collagen and may help prevent basal cell and squamous cell carcinomas, too. These are the non-melanoma skin cancers. Nothing else you can buy in a drug or department store will be as effective and powerful. Some people do experience side effects from these, including skin irritation (dryness, redness, and peeling) and an increased sensitivity to sunlight, but most people do not experience them to the point where they want to discontinue use. There are ways to lessen any potential side effects by using a lower concentration or avoiding any supersensitive areas on the skin. This is why you would start using a retinoid once or twice a week, then eventually be applying it every night.

When to consider retinoids: Because retinoids can be used for treating skin conditions, such as acne, it's not uncommon to prescribe these for young women in their teens and twenties. It's also not uncommon for women in their twenties to start using retinoids if they have had severe sun damage in their youth. But for purely antiaging effects, retinoids are frequently used by women starting in their thirties.

Q: Can products become ineffective the longer you use them?

A: Not so fast. Your skin is not likely to get used to a product's ingredients in a way that decreases its effectiveness. Many women feel that if they are not using the latest products, they are somehow missing out. If you get a rush from buying new things, you can justify the cost by convincing yourself that your old beauty products are no longer working, but it's probably all in your head. The only product that may become less effective over time is over-the-counter acne treatments, if your acne progresses and you're using a formula that is too mild. Also, don't be afraid to start using antiaging products including vitamin A derivatives in your youth. The ingredients' benefits spring eternal (that is, they won't stop working for you).

Over-the-Counter Antiaging Products

Retinoids aside, there are also a few nonprescription antiagers available that make a difference. Set a budget first to help inure you to the siren call of mega-priced elixirs, because price isn't a reliable guide. You can spend a fortune, and if money's no object and that's your pleasure, feel free. But you don't have to. Here's what works, and a couple of things that should come with the label *caveat emptor*: buyer beware.

The cheapest antiager around: a good moisturizer. Moisturizers are like aspirin: minimiracles that we take for granted. While they won't have an effect on wrinkles per se, they do help protect skin from dryness, chapping, and weathering, and keep it smooth, soft, and healthy. And a good moisturizer will do more for you than drinking twenty glasses of water per day. Drinking water does not necessarily make skin moist. If you're truly dehydrated your skin can turn dull and peaked, but it's the moisturizer applied directly to the skin that will keep water from evaporating and give your skin a healthy, dewy appearance.

Despite their long lists of ingredients, just two types do most of the work: *emollients* and *humectants*. Emollients, such as lanolin, jojoba oil, isopropyl palmitate, propylene glycol linoleate, squalene, and glycerol stearates, act as lubricants on the surface to fill in the crevices between cells ready to shed, thus helping the loose edges of dead skin cells adhere together. They help keep the skin soft, smooth, pliable. The slippery feeling you get after applying a moisturizer is most likely coming from the emollient. Humectants, on the other hand, draw water to the skin's surface, thus increasing the water content of the *epidermis*, or outer layer. If the air around you is really humid (picture yourself on a balmy, tropical island with a rainstorm descending upon you), humectants can also draw water from the atmosphere into the epidermis. Like emollients, there are dozens of humectants available for manufacturers to use in their products. Some examples include hyaluronic acid, alpha hydroxy acids, sorbitol, glycerin, propylene glycerol, urea, and sodium lactate. Heavier ingredients like silicones, mineral oil, beeswax, cocoa butter, dimethicone, petroleum, and paraffin are categorized as *occlusives*. These also increase the water content of the skin by bolstering that barrier and retarding the evaporation of water from the surface, but these ingredients are often greasy and best left for treating superdry spots or chapped lips. (Imagine lathering Vaseline all over you!) They are most effective when applied to damp skin.

Other ingredients can include *ceramides* and *collagen*. Ceramides are lipids naturally found in the skin's top layer of the epidermis, alongside other fats such as cholesterol and fatty acids. Their chief role is to keep moisture in the skin, and they have been used to treat eczema, as studies show that people with eczema have significantly fewer ceramides in their skin.

Collagen can help give the illusion of smoothness, but don't be fooled into thinking that rubbing a collagen-containing moisturizer on your face will suddenly help your skin's natural collagen. Large collagen molecules cannot penetrate the skin's deep layers, so they remain on the surface and do not have an effect on how the skin performs. (If you want a flash course on your skin's multiple layers right away, flip to chapter 6.)

It's All an Illusion

You cannot boost your own natural oil production, but you *can* repair your barrier. That will help you hold on to moisture and oil, giving you a younger-looking appearance. And when you slather on moisturizer, you help create the illusion of naturally smooth, dewy skin.

It's important to note that even though moisturizers won't necessarily affect how the skin functions at the cellular level (that is, they won't change the production level of collagen and repair of tissue damage), they are an excellent way to keep the skin hydrated, replenishing the natural moisture elements in the upper layers and bolstering the barrier function of the skin. Yes, that smooth, dewy appearance is temporary but if you moisturize frequently you keep that glow turned on. In fact, nothing over-the-counter can change the fabric of your skin. Even a surgical facelift still leaves you with the same skin; its texture and water-holding capacity remain the same. So don't sweat over the fact it's difficult to permanently alter your skin's appearance (and be wary of moisturizers that claim to treat wrinkles and use the term *antiwrinkle*). You can have a huge impact on how your skin looks just by applying topical ingredients that give it the illusion of youth. And these ingredients can help you prevent future skin damage from the environment, so you are in actuality doing more than meets the eye!

The number of moisturizers on the market today is dizzying. I don't actually tell patients, "Go look for the following ingredients," and send them off with a long list of big words. Virtually all brands will have similar ingredients. And even though most will claim to have properties that no other moisturizer has, I doubt one is truly better than the next from a scientific standpoint. It all comes down to what you like and what you think your skin likes. Finding a moisturizer is a personal choice; you can shop at your local drugstore or splurge at the department store. All I ask is that you select a scent and texture you like and a formula that has an SPF 30 or higher unless you plan to wear a separate sunscreen as well. Also look for the word *noncomedogenic*, which means it won't clog your pores. *Oil-free* may be the term used in place of *noncomedogenic*. (*Noncomedogenic* sounds technical, but it's one of those jargon vocabulary words I can't get rid of; plus, you might come across it when you read labels. Don't let it distract you; it's a very good thing to be noncomedogenic.)

Many moisturizers that have sunscreen only contain SPF 15, which is okay so long as you slather on additional protection (aim for SPF 30). There are plenty of moisturizing sunscreens out on the market that will do double duty. Eucerin's Extra-protective Moisture Lotion, for example, is a popular one (with SPF 30) that you can find at any drugstore. You can also opt to buy two moisturizers: one for your face that feels lighter and one for your body that's a little heavier. Up to you.

I'll be giving you plenty of ideas coming up shortly, as well as specifics about sunscreen in chapter 8. At the beginning of your nine-day program I'll list examples of products to consider and tell you exactly what to do.

When to start using sunscreen. As soon as possible! Encourage your kids to wear sunscreen every day, too. Even baby formulas are available, so it's never too soon. Clearly, you don't need sunscreen in your moisturizer at night. Most people would do well to moisturize twice a day—in the morning and at night. If you have dry skin, you can use a heavier cream at night. If you have combination skin, oily in some spots but dry in others, you can mix products, using a lighter moisturizer in the oily areas and a heavier one in the dry spots. But don't feel obligated to do this; go with what's easy and quick for you, and what also works well with your makeup.

Q: When it comes to basic skin care, what are the biggest beauty bargains on the planet?

A: Five things instantly go on the list.

- **Vaseline**—It's the *best* lip moisturizer. And talk about cheap! By the way, don't use any lip balms that contain phenol (Blistex does, for one). They strip the top layer off your lips. That's why you get addicted to them; they remove your natural protection.
- For body lotions: **Cetaphil Moisturizing Cream** and **Neutrogena Norwegian Formula Body Lotion.** I go to the local warehouse club and buy big tubs of Cetaphil cream or the giant pump dispenser of Norwegian Formula—they're both terrific.
- Also at the local warehouse club, I buy **Dove** or **Purpose** soap by the case. (If your skin is as touchy as mine, buy Dove in the fragrance-free or sensitive-skin formulas.) Neither of these is expensive anyway, but they're a little more than some supermarket brands, so why not buy in bulk and save the difference? They don't strip your skin of good oils.
- For sunscreens, **Neutrogena Sensitive Skin SPF 30** sunblock lotion is a world-class bargain. It contains 9.1 percent titanium dioxide, a crushed mineral that protects you instantly. (No, I'm not on Neutrogena's payroll! I just like many of their products.)
- **Safflower oil.** Yes, the kitchen oil you buy at the grocery. It's a super moisturizer, especially for gator-dry legs, and gentle enough for babies (some hospitals use it on newborns). This heart-friendly, polyunsaturated oil owes its famous skin-enriching actions to its very high linoleic acid content, a fatty acid that skin normally makes to keep its moisture level up and barrier function intact. Since our body's linoleic acid production gets sluggish as we get older (it's why older people can have brutally dry skin), safflower oil helps replace it—from the outside in! Smooth it on immediately after a bath or shower while you're still damp to seal in the moisture. (Don't overdo; it takes a bit to soak in.) You'll get a chance to try this technique during the nine-day program.

The Spin on Skin Types

Oily, dry, normal, combo? I know, it can get confusing, and is compounded by confusing skin that is oily in some spots and dry in others. There are so many moisturizers on the market now that chances are you can find one that suits all of your skin's needs. Lots of people are oily primarily in the T-zone area (forehead, nose, and the area around your mouth, including the chin). Plenty of others have combination skin that's dry in some areas and oily in others. Or they are just dry (or oily!) all over. Even those with oily skin should hydrate using a sunscreen-containing lotion in the morning, then a lightweight moisturizer at night.

The antiaging exfoliators: AHAs and BHAs. Otherwise known as *alpha hydroxy acids* and *beta hydroxy acids,* both of these smooth skin's outer surface and speed up cell turnover, which slows with age. AHAs (also called *glycolic* or *lactic* acids) are water-soluble and come from fruit and milk sugars; BHAs, such as *salicylic acid,* are oil-soluble, so they help to clean out clogged pores. BHAs are made from willow bark and sweet birch trees. In high concentrations, both AHAs and BHAs can help fade brown spots and fine wrinkles, but they also make skin extra sun sensitive, so sunscreens are mandatory when you're using them.

Although lots of products, from face washes to toners, scrubs, and masks, include AHAs, the concentration is often too low to do much. If you find a label that gives the percentage, try not to go above 8 percent. In all honesty I'm not a huge fan of AHAs and prefer my patients to use BHAs. Alpha hydroxy acids tend to be more irritating and stinging than BHAs, so I recommend experimenting with them

B Is for Better

Beta hydroxy acids are better than alpha hydroxy acids. The most common BHA is salicylic acid. Try adding a salicylic-acid-based toner to your skin-care routine. You may not need a toner every day; start with every other day or a few days a week. If you overexfoliate, you could irritate!

Skin Fact

Gentle exfoliation can help dry skin hold on to moisture.

first before loading up on a month's supply. I find that BHAs are not only less irritating, but also can be better for acne. One brand in particular that I like is Clinique, which sells a great toner made with salicylic acid, a classic BHA. (Clinique calls them *clarifying lotions*, even though they are in liquid form; they come in four different strengths. The most popular strength is 2, which is for combination skin—oily in the T-zone but dry in other areas.)

Contrary to conventional wisdom, you don't need to use these products every day, especially if you've got sensitive skin. Start by using them once every other day, or simply a couple of days per week. You can expect some initial stinging at first, but this may subside as your skin gets used to it. If it never seems to warm up to hydroxy acids, don't panic. There are other ways to trigger cell turnover, one of which is the old-fashioned way.

Manual—not chemical—exfoliants can also help do the trick of brushing away dead cells and that dull outer layer. Gentle grains like sugar, oatmeal, or small synthetic beads can be found in common exfoliating products you can use once or twice weekly, depending on the sensitivity of your skin. Exfoliation is a practice that requires experimentation. Some people can tolerate the more abrasive products while others need more gentle formulas that won't leave skin red and irritated. On the one hand, you're scrubbing away dead, dulling cells to stimulate new cell growth and reveal that healthy, fresh glow. But on the other hand, you're doing just that: semisanding your face! Finding the balance here is key.

Skin Tip

Don't schedule a facial, chemical peel, or microdermabrasion the same day as a big event. Give yourself at least a week to allow for any irritation to go away.

If you want a more aggressive approach to exfoliation, you can schedule a visit to a dermatologist for a glycolic peel or microdermabrasion. Many have medical assistants or aestheticians in their offices who do these treatments daily. Here's a quick description of how these work.

During a microdermabrasion treatment, a special machine is used to remove the outermost layer of skin cells. Some machines use tiny crystals and others have diamond-encrusted wands. Then, a vacuum applied over the skin sucks away the dead cells, revealing a brighter, smoother complexion.

Chemical peels generally entail a solution of concentrated glycolic or salicylic acid that is applied to the skin. Other peels are available that can go deeper. Your skin will be pink for several hours following such a treatment, but then will glow for days.

Q: I've always been scared to get a facial for fear that it will cause me to break out. Is it okay to get a facial that is meant to extract zits? What about organic enzyme facials, nourishing facials that use plant extracts and fruit acids?

A: First, you don't need facials or expensive products to get great skin. The key is keeping a simple, gentle, and consistent routine. That said, the pampering aspect to getting a facial definitely gets my green light, and there's nothing wrong with trying one if you've never had the experience (and please, use all the relaxing amenities available to you if you visit a day spa for your facial!). But don't ask for the triple-strength special; start with the most gentle form available to you, and don't plan your facial the same day as a big night out. You may experience some redness and tenderness, but a good facial should not irritate your skin to the point at which it triggers inflammation and acne. Ask your friends for a recommendation on a particular spa and/or trusted facialist so you don't have to choose somebody blindly.

When to start exfoliating regularly. Exfoliation is something you want to do starting in your teens, and for sure by your twenties and thirties. By the time you reach your thirties, your skin begins to thin and becomes even more vulnerable to the environment. At the same time, the natural enzymes in your skin begin to work less effectively at removing dead skin cells, so they hang on and prevent your skin from reflecting light. The result? You look ashy and gray.

While you can certainly test this in your twenties, you may want to consider scheduling a mild peel or microdermabrasion once a month when you reach your thirties. Then, in your forties, it may be time to bump up the frequency to twice a month. It will all depend on your individual skin type and texture. If exfoliation makes your skin irritated and red, don't do it as frequently or lighten up on the harshness of your methods. Remember, if you overtreat and irritate your skin, you could be setting yourself up for more skin problems.

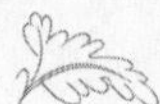

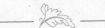

Home Kits for Microdermabrasion and Chemical Peels Beware of home kits for peels and microdermabrasion. I understand that many people rave about these, but I find they fall into one of two categories: They can be too mild to do anything (and be a total waste of your money), and they can harm you if you don't know what you are doing and you've chosen a strong product. A microdermabrasion kit won't entail machinery, but rather rubbing a high concentration of crystals onto your face to get a similar, albeit weaker, effect. Take-home chemical peels will only contain 10 to 20 percent solution, which minimizes the risk of burning, but these can still be strong enough to bother you. Gentle formulas are also available, such as ones that use lactic acid. If you have very sensitive skin and cannot tolerate these peels, try an enzyme peel made from natural fruit enzymes.

If you decide to go this route, and don't want to schedule a trial run in a dermatologist's office, then at least do a spot test underneath your forearm or in front of your ear (on the side of your face) for three nights in a row. If you don't notice any obvious irritation, you can proceed.

Antioxidants: The list of these free-radical fighters, which are added in topicals, is constantly growing and includes certain ingredients found in pomegranate, grape-seed extract, green tea, red wine, dark chocolate, coffeeberry (which comes from the fruit of the coffee plant), as well as vitamins C and E. When they work—and some, like green tea and dark chocolate, look more promising than others—they can protect skin from sunburn, inflammation, DNA damage, and skin cancers. Topical caffeine has been getting lots of attention in research circles, as it may repair UV damage and be among the strongest antioxidants around. Of course, the active ingredient—such as resveratrol in red wine and EGCG in green tea—has to be identified, extracted, and then added to a cream or other vehicle first.

The challenge for cosmetic chemists is making these ingredients stable so they are still potent when they hit your skin. I have my doubts, for example, about coenzyme Q10 (which you'll find in lots of antiaging products), because I think it's ineffective when applied to the skin, and becomes deactivated quickly. Similarly, vitamin C is very unstable and is usually deactivated in the environment quickly by light and oxygen, long before it has a chance to do anything in your skin. For this reason, I don't tell my patients to seek out topical vitamin C formulas; you have to be very careful about selecting one that allows you to make the most of that vitamin C, and that can be very hard to do (especially when faced with all those advertising claims).

One result du jour: serums, which are billed as supercharged antioxidant delivery systems. While their skin benefits aren't 100 percent proven yet, I believe in the basic science. There's growing evidence that they both prevent and treat sun damage, and quash skin-damaging oxidants from pollution, too. It takes a high concentration, as much as 90 percent polyphenols, to have an effect and so far only some of the more expensive companies specifically state the percent of antioxidants on the labels. So I tell patients that if they can fit a good antioxidant into their budget, I say go for it. It doesn't hurt to use them as an additional age-protection tactic.

When to start using antioxidants. Like sunscreen, it's never too early to start protecting yourself against the harsh environment. Women in their twenties should consider adding an antioxidant serum to their daily regimen.

Retinols. These are basically retinoids light—over-the-counter derivatives of vitamin A that are not strong enough to need a prescription. As such, they are also not strong enough to deliver the same antiaging goodies: replenishing collagen, undoing sun damage. On the plus side, they are far less likely to irritate skin than prescription-strength retinoids like Retin-A and Tazorac, and for some people they can improve wrinkles, roughness, and overall aging ever so slightly. Unlike their prescription-level counterparts, retinols are nothing to write home about—yet. New formulations are currently being tested, and I'm hoping more products soon emerge that generate better results worth spending money on. A product that has recently emerged, and that I like to mention to my patients, is called Topix Replenix Retinol Smoothing Serum. One bonus is this particular product has 90 percent green tea polyphenol extract, which helps counteract free radicals and any possible irritation in the skin. So, at least you're getting a moisturizing antioxidant serum.

Suck It Up a Little

It's nearly impossible to divorce irritation from efficacy. Products that generate the best results often come with some minor irritation, especially at the start of using them. Most people, however, get over the initial irritation and enjoy the benefits that accompany the outcome.

When to start considering the use of retinols. Most of my patients who start using retinols for antiaging effects begin in their thirties or later, as with the more powerful retinoids, but it's not unusual to suggest that a twenty-year-old who has had lots of sun exposure in her life use a night cream containing retinols or retinoids. And, by the same token, it's never too late. Women in their fifties and beyond can benefit.

Lighteners/brighteners/bleachers. Brown spots, splotches, darker areas—all are a result of hyperpigmentation, that is, too much melanin rising to your skin's surface. The problem of hyperpigmentation is a common, and quite irksome, frustration for many women of difference races. The most effective bleaching agent is hydroquinone, which is available in both 2 percent over the counter and 4 percent prescription strengths. Other options include arbutin, licorice extract, and kojic acid (but I have never seen great results from these). During pregnancy, azaleic acid is a milder alternative; it's also good for fighting acne during those nine months. Whatever you try, nothing will work for long if you don't faithfully use a broad-spectrum, high-SPF sunscreen to keep additional melanin production at bay.

Hydroquinone, while the most powerful bleaching agent, actually does not bleach the skin. It inhibits a pigment-forming enzyme so that new cells don't darken. But it has had its bad day in the spotlight, which is why it's banned in Japan, European Union countries, and Australia. In 2006, the FDA proposed removing it from its safe ingredient list for over-the-counter formulas (if it does become banned, it will still be available as a prescription). The reasons are potential carcinogenicity and a very rare side effect, called *ochronosis,* that can occur with long-term use, especially in people of color. Instead of a lightening effect in the treated area, some people experience the opposite—a darkening or bluish hue. The studies that gave hydroquinone bad press were on rodent data for ingested hydroquinone, and most doctors (including me) think it's too big a leap to say humans who use this in a topical form are at serious risk, but it is certainly possible. Most of us consume hydroquinone daily in foods such as berries, coffee, wheat, and tea.

When to consider lighteners/brighteners/bleachers. Discoloration can arise at any age, but it's most likely going to show up in women past age twenty, and especially in women of color. Discoloration can also be the result of pregnancy, birth control pills, the sun, acne, and scars. If you want to try hydroquinone, assuming it's still available to you over the counter, I consider testing it out for a few weeks. If you don't see an improvement in those weeks, stop the product and speak with your dermatologist.

Why It's So Hard to Make an Antiager That Works

Discovering powerful antiaging ingredients is one thing. Using them is quite another. For starters, getting the stuff *into* the skin, especially if it's a big molecule, isn't easy. And keeping it stable enough to do its job can be even trickier. Take *hyaluronic acid.* It's a natural skin component and a great plumper (when injected) because it's water loving. Inject it directly into the dermis and it happily fills in wrinkles for approximately four to eight months and may even spur new collagen production. If hyaluronic acid is added to a moisturizer, it won't spur new collagen but as a humectant it can add to the moisturizer's hydrating qualities. Likewise, in the test tube, vitamin C is a potent antioxidant that helps reverse UV damage, but it's also highly unstable. Take it out of a tightly controlled lab situation and put it in a bottle you open in your bathroom twice a day, exposing it to sunlight and air, and how much survives and actually winds up on your face is anybody's guess.

Two Ingredients That May Not Be Worth a Dime—Yet

The technology for beauty products changes rapidly. At this writing, I don't encourage the use of peptides and growth factors for the reasons I will discuss. But this may change as new products emerge that eliminate the problem associated with these ingredients.

Peptides. These protein fragments, composed of amino acids, are like errand runners within cells, telling them to switch various functions on or off. If you put them on fibroblasts in the deeper layers of skin, they'll set off collagen production. But there's a big *but:* Whether it's a pentapeptide or an oligopeptide, these molecules are way too big to slip through the epidermis, which is a very powerful and effective barrier. So even if they are added to a moisturizer, they're not going to have any underlying effect.

Growth factors. Skin-care products that tout ingredients like epidermal growth factor make me nervous—and should make you nervous, too. What if they stimulate growth in cells that cause cancer? If these ingredients really worked, they would have to be controlled by the FDA, because they would be considered drugs. Regardless, buyer beware: I'd keep my skin and wallet a safe distance from them.

Don't Be Fooled!

When manufacturers market a beauty product, they can make claims that are not approved by the FDA. An "effective antiaging treatment," for example, could simply mean the product is moisturizing the skin. You won't know what works for you in the antiaging category until you test a product yourself, using the old-fashioned trial and error.

the daily practice

Time is of the essence every minute of the day, even more so in the morning. I understand the need to make this routine as quick and easy as possible. Actually, the less you do, the better. Your morning and evening routines will be slightly different, but both won't take longer than it does to brush your teeth. Your body, including your skin cells, operates differently at various hours of the day. Just as your body has a predictable circadian rhythm, your skin cells follow a cyclic pattern that can be matched with an ideal treatment plan. Let's take a look at what you should be doing in the morning versus the evening. I'll help you to set this in motion on Day One.

The Morning Ritual

Your skin, as does the rest of your body, knows it needs to saddle up for the day's long battle in the elements. Skin cells go into survival mode by producing more *sebum* (the oily substance), which peaks at noon. Sebum is what delivers the antioxidant vitamin E to the skin's surface to help mitigate the effects of damaging sunlight and air pollution. The goal of your morning routine is to prepare the skin for the day and help boost its protectionist methods.

Q: My face is always shiny. Am I stuck with an oily face forever?

A: When patients complain about oily faces, one of the first things I ask about is their daily treatment regimen. If you overclean and dry out your face with excessive use of soaps, gritty scrubs, and toners (especially alcohol-based ones), you could be causing your skin to react by producing *more* oil to compensate, not less. Your genes and hormones can also be adding to this. The solution? Get your daily cleaning regimen down to basics: Use a gentle soap like Cetaphil Daily Facial Cleanser for normal to oily skin, see if you can go tonerless for a few days, and moisturize with an oil-free formula. During the day, you can blot your oily spots with blotting papers. If you still can't seem to get a handle on your oil faucet and it bothers you, consider a topical retinoid product. Retin-A, for example, has been shown to control oiliness.

First, take warm, not hot, showers and use a gentle soap or cleanser (my faves: Dove, Purpose, Cetaphil). You can use these gentle soaps on your entire body, including your face. Feel free to use a loofah or scrub on your body if you don't become irritated, but avoid using any scrubs on your face. Your hands and a light lathering of soap will do just fine.

Keep your showers short and use soap sparingly. Both hot water and soap dissolve body oils and make skin dry, which is why it's key to minimize this effect with warm water and minimal soap. Wash only the dirty parts! Skin should be clean, not dry. If you're fighting adult acne on your face or body (a topic I'll cover at length in chapter 8), use an antiacne cleanser that contains benzoyl peroxide and/or salicylic acid. Neutrogena Oil-Free Acne Wash, Clinique Acne Solutions (you can choose between the Cleansing Foam and Cleansing Bar), and Clean & Clear Advantage Acne Cleanser are all good choices. If these are too drying for

Lose the Loofah!

Don't ever use a loofah on your face; lose the facecloth, too. Use your own hands to wash your face, which won't harbor as much bacteria as an old rag that you've been using all week. If you must use a loofah, keep it below your neckline.

your face, however, just use regular soap; don't be afraid to moisturize your face even though you have acne. A face that has acne still needs to be cleansed and moisturized.

If your hair is fine or dry, like mine, wash it every other day, for the same reason—it will get parched otherwise. If you work out in the morning, but don't necessarily want to wash your hair that day, you can simply rinse your hair with warm water to get the sweat out and apply some conditioner to keep it soft (or you can use just a smidgen of shampoo and try using the conditioner before the shampoo so you help minimize the shampoo's drying effect).

When you get out of the shower, use three separate towels, one each for hair and face and body. Reserve the face towel only for your face and wash it extraoften to keep bacteria from building up—it's a simple pimple preventer.

Laser or Electrolysis?

Electrolysis is not the same thing as laser hair removal. Electrolysis uses a needle with an electrical current flowing through it that penetrates deep into the hair follicle. A laser, on the other hand, uses the energy from a laser light to zap the follicle. Which is better? Well, I prefer laser because it doesn't involve a needle, and is much faster and more efficient. But here's the caveat: A laser doesn't work well on blond or gray hair, and it's more costly.

Afterward, moisturize every inch but do your face first so residues from body lotions, which likely aren't antiacnegenic, don't get on your face and encourage a breakout. I like to use an antiacne face moisturizer (again, look for the words *oil-free* or *noncomedogenic* on the label).

In the morning, *always* use a facial moisturizer with sunscreen—please, at least SPF 30. In the summer, I switch to an SPF 50. I put it on my face, chest, forearms, hands, anything that will be exposed that day, depending on what I'm wearing. If you don't go through a tube a month, you're not using enough (the entire face needs about a teaspoonful). You may also choose to apply a cream containing antioxidants if these aren't already in your moisturizer, so you arm your face before it goes to meet the day's battle in the environment. One example of a brand that offers a well-founded product with a blend of powerful anti-

Q: I get wicked razor burn sometimes on my legs and under my arms. Is there any foolproof way to avoid this? Or treat it so it doesn't happen again? What am I doing wrong with my shaving?

A: A razor burn results when the follicles become irritated. You'll see the redness within minutes to hours. It can happen frequently if you shave too closely, too harshly, too quickly, or on skin that's not softened by the warm water enough to endure the abrasion. Almost every woman experiences razor burn at some point; avoiding it to begin with is the best medicine, since the rash can be painful. If you try to shave again too soon, it can avalanche into a series of razor burns as you continue to irritate your skin.

To treat a razor burn get yourself an over-the-counter tube of hydrocortisone (0.5 to 1 percent strength) and apply it to the affected area twice a day. Switch from regular shaving cream or gel to a hypoallergenic and fragrance-free variety; try Aveeno Ultracalming Shave Gel or Kiehl's Simply Mahvelous Legs Shave Cream (and finish it off with Kiehl's Simply Mahvelous Legs After-Shave Lotion). Alternatively, you can also go for Clinique's line of shaving products; even though they are marketed for men they can work wonders on women's legs, too! If you've been using a razor with three or more blades, decrease to a two-bladed razor.

To avoid razor burn: Use good razors, and change your blade at least once a week; shave toward the end of your shower after your skin has softened from the heat, use a shaving cream or gel, go slowly and don't push into your skin, and don't go over the same area twice. If razor burn is a persistent problem, consider laser treatment, which damages the hair follicles and prevents hair growth. Laser hair removal typically requires a series of treatments (five to seven), followed by a touch-up every six months to a year.

oxidants and sunscreen is Topix Replenix CF Anti-Photoaging Complex SPF 45. (Again, for more information on sunscreen, see chapter 8.)

Remember, choosing the right lotions (moisturizer, sunscreen, antioxidant cream, etc.) is a personal decision. Experiment with different brands to find the formulas and consistencies you like. You may not need a thick, heavy cream, for instance. If your face tends to leak oils (you get that shiny glow after a couple of hours), try a lighter moisturizer. You'll also find formulas for combination and extradry skin. Before moving on to richer formulas, just try using a bit more and see if that works.

Hair Therapy: Don't Give It the Shaft!

Virtually every woman has experienced the magic of getting a great cut or style from a salon. It can make you feel—and look—wonderful. Don't underestimate the power of great hair in topping off your looks. There are just as many hair products on the shelves as there are antiaging products. Some claim to make your hair look thicker, smoother, lighter, fluffier, shinier, and so on. Experiment with different products to find the one that you like and that your hair seems to like, too. I have very fine, straight hair so it helps to use a shampoo and conditioner for fine or thin hair, and blow out my hair with a hair dryer. Don't drive yourself nuts because there is no best product. And when you find something good, stick with it! News flash: It's a myth that you must change your shampoo and conditioner frequently so that your hair continues to respond. Here are a few other tips for those whose manes are less impressive than they were in their teens. Dealing with thinning hair can be a challenge (not to mention an emotional letdown), but thankfully there are some tricks to make the most of what you've got.

- Try an over-the-counter topical solution of 2.5 percent minoxidil, which is both the generic and chemical name for Rogaine. If you don't see results after using it twice daily for six months, give it up, and ask your physician about other options available by prescription. Remember, hair loss can have an underlying medical cause. Your doctor can test to see if you are anemic (have low iron) or have an underperforming thyroid. Other medication you may be taking and stress can also be partly to blame.

- Find a great hairstylist. Be open with him or her about your hair loss (you won't be the first person to admit it!).
- Try coloring your hair. Adding highlights can move attention away from your thinning areas. In addition, it can give your hair shaft a boost, plumping it and enriching its volume.

The Best Makeup for Your Skin

It's rare to have reactions or outbreaks from makeup products, so choose whatever makeup you like. It'd be impossible to list all the brands that make wonderful makeup, from both department stores, drugstores, and places like Sephora. *Allure* magazine keeps a Master List, which you can access online at www.allure.com/beauty/bestof if you want to know what others have voted as the best cosmetics for eyes, lips, foundation, and so on. As for me personally? I enjoy Shiseido and a line also owned by Shiseido called Clé de Peau Beauté (you can find local stores that carry this at www.cledepeau-beaute.com; they make deliciously wonderful skin-care and makeup products). Other faves include Clinique, M.A.C., and Bobbi Brown. (See the Q&A box for ideas on the best beauty splurges.) One thing to note: Maybelline routinely wins for being one of the best makers of mascara. If you've got sensitive eyes or wear contact lenses, though, and you tend to get red eye, try Almay's hypoallergenic line of mascaras designed for contact lens wearers. It will say this on the package.

Q: Minerals aren't just in food and vitamins anymore. What do you think about all the mineral-based makeups that are so popular?

A: Like most trends—though this one may last—they have both pros and cons. Here are the cons:

- Yes, minerals naturally act as a sun barrier, but the amount you get from these is likely to be significantly less than the label promises, because what people often love about them is that you don't have to use much—they are light and sheer, and it just takes a little to get the effect you want. You'd have to wear a *lot* to get an SPF 15 or higher. Don't get a false sense of sun security. It's the same thing that happens when you put only a dab of SPF 30 on your face; you need a whole teaspoonful.
- Some of these makeup lines swear they are fine to sleep in. Yes, it's probably better than falling asleep in regular makeup, but don't sleep in any makeup!
- The colors are limited and they can be both messy to use and a little tricky to control.

Here are the pros:

- They are great for people with sensitive skin. I use a mineral blush myself! No one reacts to them because there's nothing to react to: Minerals are chemically inert. And they sit right on the surface of the skin.
- They are fine for acne, too, because they are inherently noncomedogenic.
- Once you get good at using them, they are light and pretty.

Choosing whether to use mineral-based makeup is up to you. If regular, nonmineral-based makeup has suited you for years and you enjoy it, why change? Remember, there are no rules to makeup. It's a personal choice, no matter what the advertising hype.

The Cool Cucumber: Skin's Best Friend

Baggy eyes are easier to banish than dark circles. In fact, concealer is your best bet for masking those dreaded dark circles under your eyes. And for tackling eye bags, cucumbers can rescue more than those puffy undereye clouds.

Cucumbers reach their peak in July and August, so make the most of farmers' market bargains and load up with a half-dozen: three for salads and three for your skin. (You can get this vegetable any time of year, too, so no excuses!) This crunchy green vegetable is not only low in calories, it's also full of vitamins, minerals, and antioxidants that can feed your complexion inside and out. Here's how.

Refreshes and Protects: Cucumbers contain vitamin C and *caffeic acid,* two antioxidants that, when applied to the skin, help fend off wrinkles, sun damage, and more. Vitamin C helps builds collagen and elastin, those protein fibers that give skin its youthful plumpness. And caffeic acid inhibits cancer cells and protects skin cells exposed to UV radiation. No wonder some spas offer hydrating face treatments made of crushed cucumber. Home version for kitchen divas: Barely puree half a cucumber and two to three tablespoons of plain yogurt in the blender; it should be thick, not drippy. Pat all over your face and neck, stretch out for fifteen minutes or so, rinse, and relish how good your skin feels.

Deflates Puffy Peepers: Refrigerated and sliced into rounds, cucumbers fit neatly over eye sockets, where they act like delicate mini-ice packs and relieve puffy lids. One reason: Cucumbers are 90 percent water, which helps them stay chilly even on hot spots. Their cold minimizes the swelling by constricting the blood and lymph vessels that bring fluid to the eye area.

Don't Be Fooled!

The eyes don't need special treatment. Don't waste your money on expensive eye creams. The skin around your eyes may be delicate, but it doesn't need a special formula! Your regular moisturizer will do just fine.

Gets the Red Out: Cucumbers' natural anti-inflammatories calm and soothe skin reddened by rosacea or sunburn. Place thin, cold slices on the butterfly region of your face, starting around your nose and spreading out onto your cheeks—or anywhere there's redness. After a fifteen-minute lie-down, remove and apply a light moisturizer. Alternatively, try Peter Thomas Roth's Cucumber Gel Masque, one of those cult beauty products that, even at a forty-five dollars, gets raves from ordinary users.

The Nightly Prescription

Your routine at night will take a minute longer because now you've got your makeup and all the dirt and residue buildup from the day to take off. But this doesn't have to be laborious. If you washed your face in the morning, you can use the same mild cleanser such as Cetaphil liquid or a Dove bar at night so long as it removes your makeup efficiently. It helps to use a separate eye-makeup remover on both your eyes and lips (especially if you've been wearing a heavy-duty, long-lasting lipstick). One to try (and that you can pick up in just about any drugstore) is Almay Eye Makeup Remover Pads. If you've got oily skin, a foaming cleaner may be best. Cleansers with hydroxy acids (such as glycolic or salicylic acid) can help exfoliate your skin and help reduce the appearance of fine lines but again, you may not want to exfoliate every day; this is a treatment you'll want to do weekly, biweekly, or once every few days based on your personal skin needs. If you must use one to get that cool, refreshing feeling, find a gentle alcohol-free toner that won't exacerbate any dryness (one to try: Kiehl's Cucumber Herbal Alcohol-Free Toner).

> ***Skin Tip***
>
> Avoid harsh soaps. Squeaky clean often means dryness. Go for a mild, hydrating cleanser that leaves behind a layer of lipids even after you rinse. Wash just enough to remove makeup and dirt. Don't leave the bathroom with tight-feeling skin.

Use lukewarm water and be sure to work your cleanser all over: above the browline, into the hairline, and down past your jawline. Use your hands rather than a washcloth; washcloths can actually transfer pore-clogging bacteria to your face after a few uses. Pat your skin dry with a soft, clean towel. No rubbing!

Then, it's time to put on your night creams and any antiaging formulas that should be applied at night, such as retinols or prescription retinoids. When your body unwinds and relaxes during sleep, certain parts of you go into power-saving mode, while other parts turn on and go to work repairing and rejuvenating your cells. Your body's cellular (and skin!) renewal team has the

Skin Tip

Give products up to six months to work and show results.

night shift, so this is when want to equip your skin with as many nutrients and hydrating ingredients it needs to do a fine job.

Apply your antiaging products first, then your moisturizer last, unless your antiaging product doubles as a good moisturizer. You can choose to put on a heavier cream at night if you'd like, and you do not need a separate eye cream unless you find your regular moisturizer irritating to that area. Pull your hair away from your face before hitting the pillow.

And, finally, good night!

More FAQ

Q: What are the most-worth-it beauty splurges?

A: As you've probably gathered, I'm a big believer in simple, basic products. But who doesn't love a little luxurious skin treat now and then? Nobody *needs* a two-hundred-and-fifty-dollar moisturizer but, if money is no object and you love the way it looks and feels, fine. That's not my weakness, but these are:

- **Lipsticks.** They're the one makeup item I'll really splurge on because I adore the way they feel. Shiseido and Cle de Peau (which is actually part of Shiseido) are amazing—the colors and the textures—but, for me, any great lipstick is hard to resist.
- **Antioxidant treatments**, particularly the ones based on green tea or caffeine. A line I personally like is Topix Replenix. Its antioxidant Cream CF or Serum CF are caffeine enhanced *and* have 90 percent polyphenols from green tea. They cost about sixty dollars each at www.skinstore.com. I find the cream slightly more moisturizing, so it's good for dry types like me; oilier skin would be fine with the serum.
- **L'Occitane's olive-oil skin products.** Like safflower oil, olive oil is a great moisturizing skin treatment but leaves you smelling like a salad. These don't.

- **La Roche-Posay Anthelios XL 50 sunscreen.** I love them but they're definitely expensive in the U.S., if you can find them at all. I either order them online from Canadian pharmacies or coax friends who are going to Europe to pick up several tubes for me. They can be sixty dollars a tube here but, if you shop hard, twenty dollars outside the country.

Q: Which ingredients are most likely to irritate sensitive skin?

A: These are the top five, based both on my medical knowledge and on my personal experience—I'm the queen of sensitive skin. I inherited tons of good genes from my dad, but I also got his supersensitive skin. I'm allergic to everything from the adhesive on bandages to almost all fragrances. So, while I get to try almost every skin-care product that's made—which may sound dreamy to people who are more mesmerized by Sephora than Godiva—I usually react to anything that's not fragrance free. And since nonstop stress can make anyone's skin sensitive, if you suddenly react to something, check product labels for these:

- **Fragrance of any kind.** Even if it's the very last item on the ingredients list, meaning there's only a tiny amount, it can be a problem for people like me.
- **Cinnamates.** They're used in some sunscreens (where they're usually listed as *methylcinnamate*) and lipsticks. Yes, they come from cinnamon but you're not likely to have any problems with the spice, just this derivative.
- **Lanolin and mineral oil.** Lots of people react to these, although they've been around for centuries and remain fairly common ingredients in skin treatments. Lanolin is why some people have problems with Aquaphor, which otherwise is an extremely good moisturizer.
- **Helioplex.** It's a relatively new sunscreen agent that does an excellent job at blocking both UVA and UVB rays, but I'd say 99 percent of the sunscreen rashes I saw during the summer of 2007, when it really hit the market, were Helioplex related. It reminds me of the problems with PABA, which worked well but also irritated so many people that it's no longer common in sunscreens. They may find a way to solve the Helioplex reactions, though.
- **Sorbic acid.** It's used in prescription retinoid creams as a preservative, but it's a key reason that many people find them irritating at first.

If your skin reacts to one of these, it doesn't mean all the others will bother you, too, or that nothing else will! I have to be careful with nearly everything on the list, yet sometimes I can use a product with fragrance. On the other hand, propylene glycol can get to my skin. You start to figure these things out for yourself. And sometimes a whole product line won't agree with your skin, yet there's no obvious reason why. I often have patients say, "You know, I just can't wear brand X—am I crazy?" The answer is no. It's not *that* uncommon.

3

the seven healthy (free) habits for healthy skin

How to Take Six Years off Your Face Naturally

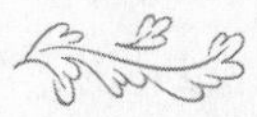

If I had to give you one word that is the root of all evils today, at least when it comes to health and beauty, it's *stress*. Not diet, not drugs, not smoking, not alcohol, not pollution or global warming, and definitely not the trans fats or fast food that infiltrate our everyday lives. The biggest beauty thief and ager of all is the stress our minds try to endure day in and day out. And I hope the tests you took in the first chapter didn't stress you out too much! I'll be taking you through the anatomy of stress and skin in later chapters. I'll also explain in depth how stress aging and the mind-beauty connection works. But I know most of you just want to get started right away with what to actually *do*.

Now that you've gotten a lesson on caring for your skin, it's time to learn what else you can do to nurture the healthiest, most vibrant skin possible from the inside out. I call these strategies the seven healthy habits for healthy skin because they are just that: habits that you form to support radiant physical beauty. All of them will help you to combat the stress that can age you six years or more. You will focus on incorporating these into your life during the nine-day program laid out for you in the next chapter.

It's really true that the best things in life are free. You don't need a million bucks to feel like a million bucks (and if you do have wads of cash . . . please, go spend it somewhere else!). There's so much you can do without spending an exorbitant amount of money, or time. In fact, a lot of what you can do right away costs close to nothing, which is why I'm dedicating most of this chapter to detailing those steps you can take, with proof on how they relate to your looks and sense of well-being.

All too often we can fall into the trap of negative thinking, telling ourselves that it costs too much to be beautiful and healthy. And I'm referring not just to monetary costs, but also to the psychological component in making an effort at instigating change in your life. It can seem scary and undoable, as if you're about to stop everything you've already been doing and start a whole new life. Not so! You get to choose which action steps to take starting today, and you can build on your program as you progress. I predict, though, that as soon as you begin to see and feel results, you will embrace more and more of my recommendations. They are not radical; they are practical and sensible. And your body and mind will love it.

Here's a sneak peek at how the nine days play out:

Day One: *Simplify.* Establish a daily skin care routine and a regular (sound) sleep schedule.

Day Two: *Relax.* Book a treatment, connect with friends, try a yoga class, and/or have sex; learn simple breathing exercises you can do daily.

Day Three: *Go green.* Get out in nature and take in your surroundings.

Day Four: *Eat clean.* Avoid fast food, fried food, and anything processed.

Day Five: *Make a move.* Establish an exercise routine.

Day Six: *Foster friendships.* Connect with friends and family in person.

Day Seven: ***Pamper yourself.*** Learn how to meditate before bedtime.

Day Eight: ***Sleep in beauty.*** Sleep in or try napping.

Day Nine: ***Reflect.*** Look back on your week.

Even though I've created the upcoming program to last nine days, it may take time for your body to response to a shift in your lifestyle, however great or small. The nine days will really be a breaking-in period for you to establish these habits forever. In fact, some of these habits can create new neuronal pathways in your body. That's right: The brain is not so hardwired as we previously thought. And neither is your skin. The moment you decide to adapt these ideas to your life is the moment you begin to make physical, neurochemical, and hormonal changes in your body for the better—ones that will support your goal of bringing out the best in your looks.

The good news is that most of these habits involve doing *less*, not more, than you usually do. If you're not sure how to get started with incorporating these practices into your life, don't panic. I'll help you do just that during the nine-day program. But I want to get you thinking about establishing these habits in your life for the long haul—not just during a nine-day pocket of time.

Remember: Even small changes can have a big impact: When you're carrying around a ton of bricks, shedding just a few can make the load more manageable, and inspire you to shed a few more.

Now, let's get to those seven healthy habits.

The Seven (Free) Habits for Healthy Skin

- Practice deep breathing
- Get active
- Beat the foods that beat you
- Focus on the good things
- Stretch out your sleep
- Take a time out
- Cuddle or have sex

practice deep breathing

A classic sign of the stress response is shallow, crazy-fast breathing. That's why the opposite—deep, slow breathing—is such an effective way to calm yourself down. It can help you halt a stress reaction, or at least control it. Plus, it shifts the body's balance of carbon dioxide to oxygen in favor of energizing oxygen. Remember, carbon dioxide is a waste product, whereas your cells and systems need a constant supply of fresh oxygen to stay alive and work efficiently. Oxygen is arguably the most vital nutrient for the body; we would die within minutes without it. The integrity of the brain, nerves, glands, and internal organs depends on oxygen, and any shortage in supply will have a profound impact on the entire body—inside and out.

There are several breathing exercises, and on Day Two you will begin experimenting with a few.

How Breathing Unwinds You and Upgrades Skin

Breathing goes far beyond just delivering life-sustaining oxygen to the body. Slow, controlled breathing in particular is the foundation for many Eastern practices that aim to return the body to a more balanced state, and one that has removed all signs of stress. Yoga, qigong, and tai chi are just a few examples of such practices, and if you've ever participated in these, then you know what it feels like when you're done. You feel relaxed, replenished, and unable to entertain the thought of an argument or other stressful situation. The world just seems right.

When you're focusing on your breathing, you're not focusing on anything else (such as your lousy boss or late babysitter). That shift in your mind helps remove stressors, bringing you to a deeper level of consciousness, a place where you can put things into perspective. And let's not forget that oxygen is required for the production of the all-important energy molecule called ATP (*adenosine triphosphate*). ATP essentially acts as the transporter for energy within cells. Your skin cells in particular require a lot of energy because they are so dynamic, engaging in all sorts of activity during the day to keep you healthy.

I should mention the lymphatic system here, too, which gets a serious boost from deep breathing. Lymph is a clear fluid filled with immune cells that moves around the body in a series of vessels. It delivers nutrients and collects cellular waste while helping to destroy pathogens, including those that can downgrade your skin health. The deeper you breathe, the more you can achieve this effect. While the heart is the pump for the vascular system, the lymphatic system has no built-in pump, so it relies on your breathing and physical movement to get around the body. It has long been known that exercise stimulates this movement of lymphatic fluid, but the role of breathing wasn't entirely recognized until scientists found a way to photograph lymph flow. This is how they observed that deep breathing causes the lymph to gush through the lymphatic vessels.

It's empowering to know that something as simple (and free) as breathing can be a powerful tool to build beauty and sustain health.

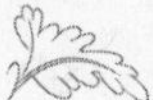

Breathe in Beauty, Breathe out Stress Your sympathetic nervous system probably works a lot of overtime. It's the part of your wiring that is sensitive to stress and anxiety, controlling your fight-or-flight response and those oft-damaging spikes in the stress hormones, cortisol and adrenaline. As chapters 5 and 6 will explain in greater detail, chronic stress burns through your body's nutrients and destabilizes your brain and hormonal chemistry. Depression, muscle tension and pain, insulin sensitivity, gastrointestinal issues, and insomnia, among scores of other conditions, are all related to a sympathetic nervous system sick and tired of working overtime. The time has come to give it a rest and bring in new shift work. What counteracts this mechanism? The *parasympathetic* nervous system, which can trigger a bona fide relaxation response. And deep breathing is the quickest means of getting these two systems to communicate, flicking the switch from high alert to low in a matter of seconds as your heart rate slows, muscles relax, and blood pressure lowers.

get active

Think about this: The stress response preps your body to leap into action. But 90 percent of the time you don't need to climb tall buildings or even dash down the street—what you need to do is *stay calm*. That's why exercise is so cathartic: It releases all that revved-up energy inside you so you actually *can* stay calm. If you can hop on a stationary bike and pedal madly for twenty to thirty minutes, great. But running the vacuum with intensity, bounding up and down the back stairs at the office, or playing fetch with Fido will accomplish the same thing, settling you down instead of leaving you pent up. At the same time, you'll boost the activity of white blood cells, increase levels of beta-endorphins, improve your mood, and get your circulation going—all good things for your skin. Beta-endorphins have immense anti-inflammatory benefits that fight your stress hormone cortisol.

I know I'm not the first person to tell you that exercise is good for you. You've heard the mantra many times before. But let me say that if there's one magic bullet for enhancing the quality of your looks, and your life in general, it's exercise. The science is well documented: Exercise fights the onset of age-related disease, lifts your spirits and sense of well-being, increases your lung capacity so you can take in more oxygen, boosts circulation to deliver nutrients to cells and skin, lowers inflammation, and, for many, is said to be the ultimate stress reducer. That healthy glow you get after a great workout (rosy cheeks indicative of the increased circulation that is nourishing all those facial cells and tissues) isn't just for show.

Quickie on Cortisol

This chief stress hormone, alongside the other major stress hormone, adrenaline, gets a lot of playtime in our modern world. In addition to getting secreted during stressful situations to assist in the well-known fight-or-flight response, cortisol also controls how your body processes carbs, fats, and proteins, and helps it to reduce inflammation. There's a good and bad side to this important hormone, depending on how much and how frequently your body releases it.

This Is Your Brain on Exercise

There's no end to the number of studies that prove the mind-beauty connection in relation to exercise. As I was writing this book another fresh study emerged clearly showing that exercise causes your brain to turn up production of certain brain chemicals known to have antidepressant effects. The researchers also found that exercise excited a gene for a nerve growth factor called VGF. VGFs are small proteins critical to the development and maintenance of nerve cells. Even more fascinating is the fact that the study brought to light thirty-three VGFs that show altered activity with exercise, the majority of which had never been identified before. It's proof that we still have more to learn about our genes and the power that our habits can have on them.

The Muscle Factor

Muscles are high-maintenance tissues, meaning they burn up a lot of calories. The more lean muscle mass you maintain as you age, the better you age, and the more calories you will burn. One feature to aging people forget about, though, is the natural decline in muscle mass and strength that occurs. Starting in our thirties, we lose an average of one-quarter of a pound of muscle each year. In terms of muscle *strength,* we lose one percent of our muscle strength every year. This picks up speed between the ages of sixty-five and seventy-five to an annual loss of 1.5 percent of our muscle strength. If you've ever been frustrated by not being able to lose weight as quickly as, say, your spouse, you can thank your lower muscle mass for that. When you do the math for this equation, you see how easy it is to fatten up automatically through the years without changing anything in your diet. If you burn 200 calories a day fewer at fifty than you did at thirty, those calories have to go somewhere if you're still consuming them.

Maintaining your muscle mass through the ages also has an aesthetic appeal. You will automatically look better because you will be toned and shapely with less sagging-and-floppy arms, and less fat.

Ideally, a well-rounded and comprehensive exercise program includes cardio work, strength training, and stretching. Each of these activities affords you unique benefits that your body needs to achieve and maintain peak performance. Cardio work, which gets your heart rate up for an extended period of time, will burn calories, lower body fat, and strengthen both your heart and lungs; strength training (use of weights or elastic bands, or even your own body weight as resistance in some cases) will keep your bones strong and prevent the loss of lean muscle mass that naturally occurs with age; and stretching will keep you flexible and less susceptible to joint pain. All three of these forms of exercise will keep your body moving and also help you to maintain good pos-

Often, Not Occasionally

To reap the most benefits of exercise, stick to a regular routine. Exercise only tames stress for up to twenty-four hours.

ture, which I have said will instantly make you look younger. The type of activity you do is not nearly as important as how often you do it, and how long you do it. Because exercise lowers stress for up to twenty-four hours, it's important to avoid being a weekend warrior and make it a goal of keeping a semidaily routine.

Don't forget that the benefits of exercise are *cumulative*. Another fact science has proven is that you don't have to sweat it out on a treadmill for a full sixty minutes. You can do ten minutes here, twenty minutes there. (Like calories, it all adds up!) Sprinkle pockets of workout times into your day—at lunch, after dinner, or in the fifteen minutes right after you get up and the house is still quiet.

Caution

I strongly encourage you to speak with your physician prior to commencing an exercise program, particularly if you have specific health issues or physical limitations to contend with or if you have not been active in a while. Your doctor can also help you gauge your fitness level and help you tailor an exercise program to your body. This will help lower your risk for injury or illness, as many people jump-start their fitness goals too quickly and wind up hurt and burned out. You must achieve a fine balance between pushing your body physically and staying attuned to its needs as you move forward.

No matter which form or type of exercise you choose to do, its positive impact on your skin and overall looks cannot be underestimated. I don't know anybody who is fit and who looks older than she should, do you? Consider all the fitness gurus in their forties, fifties, and beyond who look amazing.

Q: I haven't been active in a while, so what kind of exercise program should I start with?

A: I often recommend to my patients that they at least try walking. Not only is walking the perfect starting point for people who are not accustomed to any type of physical activity, but it's one of the most accessible forms of exercise around. You simply put on a comfortable pair of shoes (preferably ones made for walking and/or running) and step outside. You can also add as much or as little intensity to your walks as you like. This is done through speed, inclines and declines, and how long you spend walking. Try to walk thirty to forty minutes every day, but if you hate walking, don't do it! Forcing yourself to do anything you don't like is stressful. So if walking drives you crazy, but you love to dance, swim, cycle, run—you name it—you're in business.

Q: *I'm an exercise fanatic, so I'm not surprised that all those years in gyms have left me with athlete's foot. But mine is particularly annoying because it's growing underneath my toenails. My nails look thick and yellowish, with pieces of skin and nail debris under them. What can I do?*

A: These infections, called *onychomycosis*, are usually caused by a fungus but can also be caused by yeast. Those of the fungal kind, which claim about 90 percent of toenail infections, can be transmitted by direct contact or by contact with objects such as clothing, shoes, nail clippers, nail files, shower and locker room floors, and carpets. While they are not brought on by stress, they can stress you out due to their beauty-busting presence. People who get this in their fingernails tend to have a bigger problem than those who only have it on their feet. I understand how annoying it can be, and it's certainly not something you want to live with forever, much less spread to other nails in you *and* your family. Unfortunately, topical treatments usually don't do the job, but an antifungal prescription under your doctor's supervision such as Sporanox, Lamisil, or Diflucan that kills the wily beasts from the inside out can help do the trick. (And wear flip-flops in those germy public showers.)

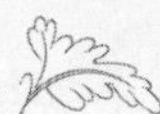

The benefits of exercise have long been reported and proven. All of the following benefits circle back to having a positive influence on your skin and the ability to maintain your youthful looks:

- increased stamina and energy
- increased flexibility
- increased blood circulation and toning of the cardiovascular system
- increased oxygen supply to cells and tissues
- more restful, sound sleep
- stress reduction
- increased muscle strength, tone, and endurance
- release of brain chemicals called endorphins, which act as natural pain relievers
- decreased food cravings
- decreased blood sugar levels, and risk for diabetes
- weight distribution and maintenance
- increased self-esteem and sense of well-being

A bit of trivia: The classic *runner's high*—the state of euphoria associated with prolonged exercise—is no longer explained solely by the adrenaline and endorphin hypothesis. Scientists now believe that the physical and psychological well-being (plus reduced anxiety, time distortion, and enhanced sensory perception) experienced by many endurance athletes is due to the exercise-induced activation of *cannabinoids*—lipids, in fact, in the body whose actions resemble those of the active ingredients of cannabis (marijuana). These cannabinoids can suppress pain at peripheral sites as well as centrally (crossing the blood-brain barrier); they inhibit swelling and inflammation; and dilate blood vessels and make breathing easier. The phenomenon of exercise addiction is largely due to these powerful chemicals naturally produced in the body.

beat the foods that beat you

Eating a box of chocolates or a pint of Ben & Jerry's when you're stressed (or just sad, frustrated, angry, and moody—all of which the body can interpret as being stressed) has its reasoning. Stress makes most of us hungry. I'll be going into more detail about the food-mood connection, plus food's connection to your skin and overall appearance, in chapter 7, but I want to introduce a few ideas here to get you thinking.

In brief, when stress hits, cortisol tells our brains that we are hungry, so we then seek out a meal. Unfortunately, cortisol's message to our brain also says we want to eat sugary, fatty foods—all the wrong foods for stopping the cycle. Rich, sugary foods don't do much for us but contribute to insulin swings, poor blood-sugar balance, as well as extra pounds, potbellies, and worse moods. What's more, the usual culprits—ice cream, cookies, Snickers bars—register in our brain's reward center in ways that make us crave them even more. During the nine-day program you're going to use the two strategies that follow to reduce the magnetic pull of these foods.

- **First, eat lots more lean protein.** This will give you more energy and fight hunger pangs, which can play games with your moods. Protein is key to mood stability, due to its effect on maintaining a healthy blood-sugar balance, which in turn keeps certain hormones like insulin in check. Carbohydrates, especially low-quality ones, aren't nearly as sustaining as good-quality proteins, such as fish, eggs, low-fat dairy, poultry, and even walnuts. Proteins are required for growing hair and nails, and they are the building blocks for enzymes and hormones, including the ones that participate in keeping you glowing beautiful.

- **Second, write down the top five guilty treats you tend to reach for when you're stressed.** Flamin' Hot Cheetos, Chunky Monkey, chips, cookies, M&Ms, whatever. Then, don't eliminate them entirely. However, when you do succumb, eat only half of what you normally would. Or less: Sometimes a bite or two will satisfy you. That's it—an easy step toward reducing your stress, steadying your weight, and shrinking your belly.

1 ____

2 ____

3 ____

4 ____

5 ____

Why are you doing this? This will help you begin to take control of your sugary portions. This isn't about deprivation, but about finding a healthy balance that will support, rather than take away from, your beauty.

focus on the good things

If you feel buoyant and upbeat, you're far less likely to start clenching your jaw. Here's an easy way to raise your happiness quotient at home, as first recommended by Martin Seligman, PhD, the scientist who inspired psychologists to investigate happiness and positive emotions.

Find a notebook or journal you particularly like—buy one with a beautiful cover or special paper if that encourages you to use it. Every night, write down three things that went well that day and why. For instance, a dinner you made that was delicious, a productive office meeting that solved a heap of problems, or a heart-to-heart with your sister that was open, honest, and caring. It may also help to keep a gratitude list; this is where you list the things for which you are truly grateful. They can be specific things like the time you spent that day with your mom, or general notes like being grateful for your children. You may find some overlap between these two lists, and that's okay. The point is to focus on the positive—on the events, people, and experiences that you appreciate and that bring you joy.

This exercise may even inspire you to turn a negative into a positive just by reshaping your attitude. For example, let's say you had a really bad day and an argument at work with a co-worker resulted in a reprimand from your boss. You have every right to be stressed and frustrated. What if you could turn that moment around by seeing its positive outcomes? What if you could see that it gave you an experience you needed to improve, to self-reflect, and to move forward? It may have been a hard lesson, but a lesson nonetheless. You can express gratitude for getting through that day, and look forward to the next one.

When you're stressed, it's easy to get caught up in thinking about what you're doing wrong. It's also very easy for the mind to exaggerate and distort the magnitude and significance of bad things that happen, and the speed with which you need to remedy them. If you don't know what I mean, then consider the last time a worry kept you up at night thinking about it like a hamster on a mill. If you were to take that worry and reassess it the next morning or afternoon, I bet it wouldn't be as big a deal as you thought while staring at the clock until two in the morning. Anxieties can quickly turn relatively harmless negative occurrences into utter catastrophes.

For this very reason, cognitive behavior therapy (CBT) is very useful in psychology. In fact, studies have shown CBT can be more effective than sleeping pills for insomniacs, underscoring just how powerful thoughts can be. As its name implies, CBT is one part cognitive and one part behavioral. The cognitive portion of CBT is about identifying, challenging, and changing the ways of thinking that leave you stressed and overanalyzing the severity of the stressor. When your mind is consumed by irritating thoughts, chances are you're fueling your own fire with a distorted, stress-inducing behavior (and the release of that cortisol won't help, either). In other words, your worries are minor, but are getting too much attention. If you could counter those negative thoughts with a positive one related to the problem, the worry would disappear.

Transforming negative thoughts takes practice. It's what CBT therapists are trained to teach. However, you can at least start by keeping a journal that records the good things that happen. It will shift the focus to what you're doing right, and that can put a brake on the stressful, negative chatter that often goes on in your head. You can do a version of this with kids, too. Every night at dinner, I ask my son and daughter to tell me the best thing about their day. It gets them to forget about anything negative that may have happened, reinforcing that the good deserves at least as much attention as the bad.

Try keeping up your journal after the program; it can work indefinitely.

stretch out your sleep

Sleep is free cosmetic medicine, pure and simple. When people ask me what's the one thing that will make the biggest improvement in how a stressed-out person looks, I say sleep. Nothing exacerbates stress and a haggard appearance like exhaustion. As you may be able to attest from experience, sleep deprivation can make you cranky, depressed, and negative. It can make you overeat, overcaffeinate, and ditch workouts because you're just too tired. How much sleep should you get? Although seven to eight hours a night is the average goal, don't ever assume you're average. If you don't wake up refreshed or you feel sleepy during the day, you probably need more pillow time, even if you're getting seven hours or more. I understand that sleep can be difficult to get, but make it a goal to do what you can to sleep the amount you need to feel alive the next day—all day. During the nine-day program your first step will be to make sleep a priority, and I'm going to help you do that starting on Day One.

The Supremacy of Sleep

Today, sleep medicine is a highly regarded field of study that continues to provide insights into the power of sleep in the support of health and beauty, as well as longevity. Just about every system in the body, including your innerbeautification capabilities, is affected by the quality and amount of sleep you get each night.

One underappreciated aspect to sleep that is especially influential to our sense of well-being is its control of our hormonal cycles. So much of our *circadian rhythm*—the cycles our bodies experience throughout the twenty-four-hour day—revolves around our sleep habits. A healthy day/night cycle is tied into our normal hormonal secretion patterns, from those associated with our eating habits to those that relate to stress and cellular recovery. Cortisol, for example, should be highest in the morning and progressively decrease throughout the day, with the lowest levels occurring after eleven at night. With (hopefully) low evening cortisol levels, melatonin levels rise. This is the hormone that tells you it's time to sleep; it helps regulate your twenty-four-hour circadian rhythm. Once released, it slows body function, lowers blood pressure, and, in turn, core body temperature so you're prepared to sleep. Higher melatonin levels will allow for more deep sleep, which helps maintain healthy levels of growth hormone, thyroid hormone, and male and female sex hormones. All good things for keeping up appearances. Let's not forget that proper circulation in your facial skin gives your face color. Rosy cheeks after being in the cold, after you exercise, or even after feeling deep embarrassment, are the direct result of facial blood circulation. And you don't get that without adequate sleep.

Sleep deprivation is depriving you of being slim and trim. Growth hormone (GH) does more than just stimulate growth and cell reproduction; it also refreshes cells during the night when you're sleeping, and is a powerful player in your ability to maintain an ideal weight. GH effectively tells your cells to slow up on using carbs for energy and asks them to use *fat* instead. But you can't get an ample supply of GH unless you're getting your Zs. GH prefers to come out at night. As soon as you hit deep sleep, about twenty to thirty minutes after you first close your eyes, and then a couple of more times throughout the night in your sleep cycle, your pituitary releases high levels of GH, the most it's going to secrete in twenty-four hours. So, without that sleep, GH stays locked up in the pituitary, which negatively affects your proportions of fat to muscle. Over time, low GH levels are associated with high fat and low lean muscle—not to mention old eyes and that nagging, chronic, not-so-fresh look and feeling. Let GH loose by getting restful sleep.

Are you a lark or an owl? Just ask your skin cells. Do you like to get up with the chirping birds in the early morning hours or stay up late enough to hear those birds' first callings of the day? In early 2008, researchers learned that you can look at your skin cell genes to find out (in case you didn't already know). Your preference for rising early or late actually is encoded in your genes, including those found in skin cells. And scientists have engineered a way to observe and measure individual clocks in human skin cells. How? After taking skin samples from volunteers, German scientists inserted into each cell a gene that lights up in ultraviolet light when the cell is metabolically most active. The gene allowed the scientists to follow the circadian rhythm of the cells as they changed over a twenty-four-hour period. In essence, they were able to identify and track skin cells' built-in timing mechanism set by the central biological clock of the body. This is possible because most cell types have a genetic imprint of a person's unique circadian physiology. Science is still trying to understand completely how our body clocks work, and even how many body clocks we have, but it's amazing to think our skin cells can hold so much information. Later on, I'll be explaining how skin acts like the brain's twin in many ways.

The Cycles of Life

Everyone has a biological, internal, clock called a *circadian rhythm* (yes, even men can say they have a biological clock). It's the patterns of repeated activity associated with the environmental cycles of day and night—rhythms that repeat roughly every twenty-four hours. Examples include the sleep-wake cycle, the ebb and flood of hormones, the rise and fall of body temperature, and other subtle rhythms that mesh with the twenty-four-hour solar day. When your rhythm is not in sync with the twenty-four-hour solar day, you will feel (and probably look) it. Anyone who has traveled across time zones and felt off-kilter for a few days can understand this.

Q: I frown upon people who get seven or more hours of sleep a night. I think sleep is a luxury; what's the big deal? If I'm okay on five hours, is that enough for me?

A: Everyone has a different sleep need. The eight-hour rule is general, and not necessarily for those who can feel and actually be fully refreshed on fewer hours; those who don't physically need at least seven or eight hours are known as short sleepers, but they are not the majority of the population. You could be fooling yourself to think you can get by on just four hours a night, especially in the long term. Sleep is not a luxury.

In addition to seeking better, more beautiful skin, if you have been struggling to lose weight, you might want to check your sleep habits. The two digestive hormones that hold the remote control to your feelings of hunger and appetite are *ghrelin* and *leptin*. As with many hormones, these two are paired but have opposing functions. One says Go and the other says Stop. Ghrelin (your go hormone) gets secreted by the stomach when it's empty and increases your appetite. It sends a message to your brain that you need to eat. When your stomach is full, fat cells usher out the other hormone, leptin, so your brain gets the message that you are full and need to stop eating. And how do these hormones tie into sleep and your looks?

A bad night's sleep, or just not enough sleep, creates an imbalance of both ghrelin and leptin. Studies now prove that when people are allowed just four hours of sleep a night for two nights, they experience a 20 percent drop in leptin and an increase in ghrelin. They also have a marked increase (about 24 percent) in hunger and appetite. And what do they gravitate toward? Calorie-dense, high-carbohydrate foods like sweets, salty snacks, and starchy foods. Sleep loss essentially disconnects your brain from your stomach, leading to mindless eating. It deceives your body into believing it's hungry when it's not, and it also tricks you into craving foods that can sabotage a healthy diet.

In addition to your sleep habits, your environment, dietary habits, exercise patterns, personal stress levels, and your genetics may also influence the production of leptin and ghrelin. One thing is certain: This just goes to show you how many biological factors contribute to your behavior, which in turn influences how you feel about what you do (or not do). Poor sleep catches up to most people. It also sets people up for entering a vicious cycle whereby they plunge into deeper sleep deprivation (and reel from its numerous negative effects), and avoid healthy behavior that can counter the bad mood, such as exercise and eating right. So, even if you say you're okay on five hours, you should take a good look at your sleep habits if you are unhappy with your looks, and your weight. See what happens when you force yourself to get more sleep. You just might force yourself to lose unwanted weight and achieve a more beautiful you.

take a time-out

For most of us, life is so hyperscheduled, speedy, and "on" that we never do absolutely nothing. It's rare to set aside time to simply *be*—no agenda, no demands, no plan. (Just like a real vacation.) Find a comfortable, quiet spot to sit for ten to fifteen minutes every day, stop all your hustling and bustling . . . and simply, by yourself, be still. Slowing down in this way, if you do it every day, helps create a sense of spaciousness in your life, a break in the old routine that can open the door to new perceptions, new solutions to old problems, new possibilities. It gives your brain, your psyche, your whole being a break. Like one long peaceful sigh.

Alternatively, meditate. Instead, think of it as entering a deeply restful sleep while being fully awake, a superrelaxed state. That's what meditation is really like. Unfortunately, many people have the wrong idea about it ("I'm not seeking enlightenment; I have enough to worry about"). Once you've put a little private time for yourself on the agenda, meditation can become a valuable stress tool. It's not tricky to learn or to do, and takes only fifteen to thirty minutes per day. On Day Seven, I'll guide you through an exercise that will help you reach a meditative state.

There is lots of research explaining why it works, one reason being that it returns the brain to more primitive state, where we are less likely to hear the noise from our usual judgmental and analytical selves. Before humans evolved into complex, critically thinking beings, our brains were a bit less complicated.

We knew how to find food, water, and socialize, but we would have had a harder time with calculus and intricate planning (like your next vacation with the kids). Then we grew an outer neocortex, which added one more layer to our brains, so we could problem solve better and think more like Einstein. With the yin of this more advanced human brain and a greater capacity to think came the yang of its disadvantage: We could be overly critical and superjudgmental to the point we drive ourselves crazy, which is where the practice of meditation comes into play.

The practice casts the human brain back to its preneocortex state, allowing us to be freed of our analytical selves. In this blissful state, one is aware of senses, feelings, and state of mind, without the negativity.

From a scientific standpoint, researchers are beginning to understand how meditation affects the aging process. In 2005, researchers at Massachusetts General Hospital published an imaging study showing that particular areas of the cerebral cortex were thicker in people who frequently meditated. These areas are involved with attention and sensory processing, including the prefrontal cortex, used for planning complicated cognitive behaviors. This study showed why meditation can promote a relaxed state. Meditators shift their brain activity to different areas of the cortex. That is, brain waves in the right frontal cortex, which is a stress center, move to the calmer left frontal cortex. This shifting of brain activity to areas associated with relaxation explains why they are calmer and happier after a meditative state.

Scientists have not figured out the relationship between the thickening of the cortex and better cognitive abilities (just because you have a thicker brain doesn't mean you are more intelligent), but it's clear the aging process naturally causes a thinning of the cortex. To find that older meditators maintain their cerebral thickness in certain areas of the cortex that would otherwise have thinned over time is pretty remarkable. It appears that meditation is truly exercise for the brain, as if it helps grow stronger muscles in the areas used. It is often said that as we age, learning new skills and challenging our brains with activities like crossword puzzles helps keep our mental faculties intact and sharp. Given this new knowledge about the brain on meditation, we see how we can practice awareness—we can drop stress and focus on the here and the now without including those mental antics that pervade our everyday lives—and our brains will have a physical response that boosts our wellness. As with deep breathing, it's empowering to know that you can become proficient in a skill that could do more for your well-being than any other skill you learned in school.

Brainy Workout
Meditating is like exercise for your brain.

cuddle or have sex

What's love got to do with it? Of course you know that sex does a body good. If it didn't, then it wouldn't make us feel so fantastic and crave the next session. That's right: For once something that feels good *is* actually good for us. Sex makes us happy, and great sex in a loving, intimate relationship makes us happier. Soft, healthy skin is quite sexy on its own. But there is lots more than that going on here. For starters, sex is one of the world's best stress releasers, which means it doubles as a terrific skin treatment. The science behind the skin-sex connection is absolutely titillating, at least for science geeks, who will appreciate the stress-reducing hormonal magic that sex brings to the body. Yes, as with most everything else that we've been talking about, it all comes down to hormones—those chemical messengers that dictate how we feel.

When you're making love, all kinds of age-defying, beauty-promoting events happen as three seductive hormones spill out of the brain.

- Beta-endorphin, a natural opiate produced in the hypothalamus and in the brainstem, washes all through you, contributing to that delicious high you feel. This is the same hormone that diminishes pain levels.
- Prolactin increases give you that relaxing, tension-zapping, post-coital "ahhhhhhh." Prolactin is a chemical messenger responsible for more

than 300 functions, most of which are related in one way or another to fertility and lactation.

- Oxytocin levels also rise, promoting feelings of affection and triggering that nurturing instinct.

Exactly how these hormones affect sexual desire, arousal, and pleasure is an active area of research, but what is known so far is that all three hormones are released during orgasm and the net effect is satisfaction and contentment. And it's no surprise that your relaxed state of mind and body allows you to fall asleep rather quickly. Getting all sweaty has direct skin pluses, too, as it bathes your whole body in skin-softening oils, giving you that postcoitus afterglow.

The message, in short: Sex makes you look good and feel good. So do masturbation and just cuddling and kissing. But you know that from experience. Intimate touching releases soothing oxytocin. You burn eight to twelve calories every second you spend kissing; plus, since about thirty muscles are stimulated when you pucker up, circulation to your face gets pumped. That could explain the glow of love, and it can't hurt.

Q: *Sex for me can be a struggle because I'm embarrassed by my stretch marks. I developed pretty quickly during puberty and have been left with ugly, squiggly marks on my breasts. Now that I've had children, I have more stretch marks on my belly and around my hips. Anything I can do in my daily routine to get rid of them?*

A: Stretch marks are incredibly common among growing teens and pregnant women. In fact, about 70 percent of women get their first set in their teens from growth spurts; changes in breast size and fluctuations in weight can also cause new marks to form. Women in their thirties can have marks left over from their teens, and acquire more with pregnancy. If you have children later in life, your skin is less resilient and has more difficulty making collagen, so it doesn't bounce back as easily. The key here is to try not to gain more than the recommended twenty-five to thirty-five pounds during pregnancy.

Don't be embarrassed by your marks; you are not the only one who has them and I'm sure you are more aware of them and bothered by them than anybody else, your partner included. New marks are often red and can be itchy, and there are great treatments to remove the redness, including lasers and prescription topical retinoids (e.g., Retin-A). Pregnant women, however, cannot use retinoids, and may try an oatmeal-based cream as an alternative. Once stretch marks have faded to skin color or paler, time will help fade them, but there is currently no definitive treatment to remove the marks (and no great topical solution, either). A series of laser treatments can help, as can keeping the area supple and moisturized. Self-tanners help to mask them, and waterproof makeup will cover them up for a day at the beach.

4

nine days to a younger-looking (and feeling) you

The Five Stress Profiles and Your Program Day by Day

Welcome to your nine-day program. Let's see how just nine days can make a difference in how you look and feel. Each day presents a new focal point that you will then maintain throughout the remaining days, and hopefully for life. This is a cumulative program that progresses each and every day. So, even though you will center on your sleep habits on Day One for example, you will need to keep that focus going so when you later turn your attention to your diet choices (Day Four) you haven't let your sleep fall into the abyss.

In the next nine days, you are going to perform little shifts in the way you take care of yourself, plan your day, and prepare for the next day. I'll start by helping you identify which stress profile you match, so you can tailor the general program to your individual needs. Most of us have one weakness that overshadows the rest, whether it's not scheduling exercise or a time-out, or not getting to bed at a decent hour.

If you have already picked up on a few healthy habits and successfully implemented the ideas I've already given in the previous chapters, congratulations. You are ahead of the game and can use these next nine days to master those skills and build upon your beauty regimen. For those who have merely started thinking about making the changes, and haven't really hit *go* yet, here is where you'll find the structure you likely need to live out the plan. I'm going to give you step-by-step instructions, plus guidance through each day.

While you can certainly start this program on any day of the week, it helps to begin on a Saturday, so that you can bookend the nine days with two weekends. Start a journal if that suits your personality, and record how you feel as you progress and what techniques you like or dislike. It also helps to look ahead; read through this chapter and take note of things you may want to schedule or purchase a few days in advance. For example, if you choose to do a massage on Wednesday, plan that ahead of time. You'll find that Day Six calls for time with family and friends, so you may want to hop on the phone tonight and see who is available that night to meet you for dinner or come over. I'll also be giving you a Beauty Bonus every day, which is an additional suggestion relating directly to your skin health, which you can choose to incorporate into your day.

Bear in mind that some of these lifestyle modifications you'll be making have biological consequences. And none of these shifts becomes routine or automatic overnight. Hence the need to keep up your newly formed habits as best you can over several weeks (even after these nine days) as your body continues to adjust and respond. This is especially true for habits such as getting more active with exercise, and being more careful about how you fuel up at meals. Let these nine days be the beginning of a longer journey that will reward you time and time again with a youthful appearance and more energy, as you continue to practice these habits long into the future. This is your starting point—you are setting a course for success.

If you follow this program diligently, I guarantee that you'll begin to see a whole new you at the finish line looking back in the mirror. However, let me be clear: This can be one of the harder things you have ever done. Why? Because you're going against ingrained habits that took years to create and could take a while to break. You've been conditioned to act a certain way, and reconditioning those habits takes time, effort, and patience. Remember, do not be discouraged if you don't complete the nine days perfectly; if you cannot keep up and prefer to go a little slower, spreading out your program over the course of a longer time frame is perfectly fine. You can choose to create a nine-*week* program instead, stretching each day's new focal point over the course of a week. Just don't use that allowance as an excuse not to take action today!

Q: Who will benefit most from these nine days?

A: Ironically, the people who will shed the most years are the ones who are in the worst stress shape and have been neglecting their skin (often along with everything else). It's amazing what some R&R, a regular cleanse-and-moisturize routine, several days of healthy eating, enough sleep, and a daily walk can do. It's so simple but it's *so* transforming, physically and psychologically.

how to tailor this program to your unique stress profile

I have found that there are typically five types of stress profiles, and you can certainly have characteristics of more than one. Below are five checkboxes, each with questions that will help you to pinpoint your stress profile. Don't worry about checking more than one box, but see if you can relate to one of these people more so than the others. This miniquiz will identify your biggest issues and help you to personalize the program to your life. Following the quiz are recommendations specific to each type. You can read through them all if you like, using a highlighter to mark anything that resonates with you. Then, as you begin the nine-day program pay particular attention to what you highlighted and the suggestions specific to your profile. Some of these ideas will be specifically recommended during the program, regardless of your individual stress type.

The Stress Profile Quiz: What Is Your Number One Beauty Thief?

- Do you toss and turn most nights, then wake up feeling like a train wreck? Do you have trouble falling asleep and staying asleep?

  If you answer Yes, then Profile One is for you.

- Do you burn the candle at both ends? Are you overloaded with To Dos, overworked, and overbooked socially?

  If you answer Yes, then Profile Two is for you.

- Are you going through an emotional rough patch right now and feel like your self-esteem and confidence are at an all-time low?

  If you answer Yes, then Profile Three is for you.

- Are you recovering from a tragic or unwanted (and probably unexpected) event in your life? Do you worry that you won't get back to any semblance of normalcy, and could even spiral into a full-blown depression?

  If you answer Yes, then Profile Four is for you.

- Do you feel stuck in a bad rut? Did you pick up this book because you need to break a vicious cycle of unhealthy habits that robs your looks and energy . . . but you don't know where to start?

  If you answer Yes, then Profile Five is for you.

Profile One: The Seriously Sleep Deprived

Maybe you are menopausal or close to it, with night sweats that drench and wake you repeatedly. Or maybe you are a first-time mom adjusting to a new baby. Or maybe you find yourself paying bills at two in the morning because twenty-four hours just isn't enough for work, teenagers, the laundry, PTA meetings. . . . Or perhaps you can't turn off your mind and endless to-do lists keep you awake. Whatever the cause, you've got a sleep deficit that's outstripped the national debt. And worrying about being tired keeps you awake!

Well, rest assured (pun intended) that you're not alone. Americans get nearly an hour less sleep per day than we did forty years ago. Juggling work and family life seems to be the primary sleep robber. People in a regular nine-to-five routine who clock an *extra* ninety minutes a day on the job are more likely to be among those who get only four-and-a-half hours of snooze time per night, according to a recent study—that's not even close to what the average person needs! No wonder so many people roam around like the walking dead during the day, alternating endless cups of coffee with cans of Diet Coke.

I'm actually a fan of caffeine in reasonable amounts. It's rich in antioxidants and good for your skin, brain, and most of your body. Start living on the stuff, however, and it can unravel a healthy sleep pattern, keeping you up later and later, so you need to drink more to stay awake the next day, and the next. It's a great business model for Starbucks and Coca-Cola, though. Buy stock in them and you'll probably sleep better.

The trouble with running up sleep shortages day after day is that it may not be physically possible to make up the loss. What's more, when sleep is skimpy, your cortisol levels don't drop as much as they're supposed to at night, and growth hormone doesn't rise as much as it should, undermining muscle strength. Remember, you need a daily dose of growth hormone, which gets secreted during deep sleep, to refresh your cells and prepare you for the next day. It not only stimulates cellular growth and reproduction, but it also has strong anti-inflammatory, antifat, and anticortisol effects—all good things for beauty (not to mention weight loss!). I'll be explaining how this happens in chapters 5 and 6 but for now put restful sleep on your agenda and use these nine days to spend more time in the sack. Here's how.

Don't take your to-do list to bed. Write down the next day's list early in the evening and stick it in your bag or on the fridge. Then you won't start anxiously making mental notes the minute your head hits the pillow.

Take something. Sometimes, to kick insomnia and get back on a better sleep cycle, all you need is to break the pattern. My cheap, supersimple, method: Take an antihistamine 30 minutes before bed (regular Benadryl—not a nondrowsy formula!—works fine) for one to three nights. Antihistamines make many people sleepy. No prescription needed.

Alternatively, try valerian herbal tea or the combo of chamomile and valerian in Celestial Seasonings Sleepytime Extra Wellness Tea. It definitely helps some people. Others swear that melatonin, the sleep-regulating hormone you can find now in a supplement form over the counter, helps them, but I'm not a fan. The amount in different products can vary wildly, despite what the labels say. It may not work for you, and its long-term safety has yet to be determined. (It's also highly unlikely that you have a melatonin deficiency; you simply need to establish better sleep habits.) I'd rather see you sleep according to your own body's clock and rely on your own production of natural melatonin. If your body clock is off, try getting some natural morning sunlight on you, do some exercise during the day, don't stay up until the wee hours of the morning cleaning house, and set aside time to wind down before bedtime.

Try a bedtime snack. The best bedtime snack is one that has both complex carbohydrates and a little protein, plus some calcium. Calcium helps the brain use the amino acid tryptophan to manufacture melatonin. This explains why dairy products, which contain both tryptophan and calcium, are one of the top sleep-inducing foods. And by combining carbohydrate together with a small amount of protein, your brain produces *serotonin*, the pleasure hormone with strong ties to mood.

Snacks to Attack Insomnia

Trip up your wakefulness and doze off with these handy bedtime snacks (stay within 200 calories and eat about an hour before bedtime):

The classic PB&J (go easy on the PB, and try it on a rice cake); top off with a glass of low-fat or skim milk.

A banana with one teaspoon nut butter of your choice.

A small bowl of whole grain cereal with low-fat or skim milk.

Fruit and cottage cheese.

Whole wheat crackers and goat cheese.

A homemade oatmeal raisin cookie with low-fat or skim milk.

Get out of the bedroom. We all think that if we lie in bed long enough, sleep *will* come. Instead, our minds tend to get busier and our muscles tenser as we stress over being awake. Give it a rest. If you can't get to sleep within twenty minutes, slip out of bed and go to a safe haven—a place that's comfy, has dim lighting, and no distractions. Just sit comfortably. Or do your breathing exercises. Or read. No e-mail, television, or other electronics, though. The point is to give your mind-body a respite from trying so hard to nod off. After twenty minutes or so, go back to bed and see what happens when you're more relaxed. Repeat once or twice if necessary.

Make like a corpse. Assuming the yoga corpse pose (*savasana*) is, well, a little like playing dead. Basically, you lie on your back on a cushioned surface, legs slightly rotated out, arms at your sides but not touching your body, palms up. Then slowly s-i-n-k into the pose, breathing naturally and letting your whole body go limp. Stay in this position for a few minutes, or for as long as you like.

R-e-l-a-x. Progressive relaxation, an effective technique that's been used since the 1930s, couldn't be simpler. It's also worked for me ever since I was a homesick kid at sleepaway camp for the first time and couldn't sleep at all. A counselor taught it to me and I still use it when I need to. What to do: Stretch out in bed and, one by one, squeeze and release all the muscles in your body, starting with your scalp and working down to your toes. Ironically, tightly tensing up your muscles before relaxing them helps them relax more than just plain relaxing them.

Let scent send you to sleep. Aromas widely considered to be relaxing are rose, lavender, vanilla, and lemongrass, but different ones work for different people (some people find lavender stimulating). If one calms you, keep a sachet near your pillow at night to whiff at will, or use a scented hand lotion.

Profile Two: The Overscheduled

Many people who fit this profile are trying to do too much, day and night. You're working long, long hours to get your career in high gear, then blowing off steam late at night, trying to meet people at smoky after-hours clubs or late-night bars. What with proving yourself on the job, struggling to get a romantic relationship going, and losing sleep over both, you're ripe for burnout. And maybe breakouts, too—a nonstop lifestyle can suddenly produce a bumper crop of pimples. Some suggestions follow.

Wean Yourself from Work

How do you do this? By setting up boundaries and sticking to them, just as you keep to brushing your teeth and hair every day. Choose a time each day after which you will not do any more work. Make sure you give yourself at least one day over the weekend to goof off (no work!), whether it's by yourself or with family.

Blow out the flame. If you're truly burning the candle at both ends, you need to stop and evaluate why. Are you working sixteen-hour days? Or are you staying out late with friends to cut loose and enjoy the fruits of your labor?

If it's wall-to-wall work, you've got to take charge. It might mean a long talk with your boss or, if things are really out of hand, even switching jobs. Or it might mean you need to just stop being such a workaholic and do less.

On the flip side is our yearning to take a break by doing something exhausting. In the case of a lot of end-to-end candle burners, we party hard, drink, smoke, and stay out way past our bedtime. My advice here isn't not to have fun. On the contrary! But when you need a break, take a *break*. Six hours at Club All Night Long probably isn't it, no matter how cute the suits at the bar are.

Get a dose of morning light. Our body clocks don't exactly match the day's twenty-four-hour-day clock, which makes us want to sleep twelve minutes longer every day and stay up later every night. But you probably don't sleep later but do stay up later . . . no wonder you're wiped. What helps? Getting out of bed at the same time every morning and sitting in a sunny spot for breakfast, or exercising outdoors, or just turning on lots of lights. A dose of brightness in the morning helps synch up your internal clock with the twenty-four-hour day. Which also helps you get on regular, saner schedule.

Turn off the cell phone and PDA. More and more we're growing into a culture addicted to our BlackBerries (there's a reason they were instantly nicknamed CrackBerries). The flickering, hypnotic light from their tiny screens will arouse your brain and cut into your sleep time. Put away your electronics at least an hour before you hit the hay, if not earlier. Otherwise, you'll never get a truly restful night's sleep. (True confessions: I know about this—I've been there!)

Tell yourself how well you're doing. Even if it feels silly, give yourself a morning pep talk while you're in front of the mirror. Say a few positive affirmations, such as "I'm going to have a fabulous day; I'm beautiful and healthy, and it's up to me to make great things happen; I'm grateful for this life and I'm doing terrific." Note how well you're coping with whatever pressure you're under. Even if you don't quite believe yourself, it's still effective. Research has shown that over time, a daily rah-rah builds resilience, which can fortify you against stress.

Prep yourself. Take stock of your coming day. Note the pitfalls: the two-hour parent-teacher night that tends to last three; the regular Thursday staff meeting; the eighty-five unanswered e-mails that could consume the entire morning. Every day has its molehills, but if you're prepared and limit the time you give them, they won't turn into mountains.

Book a massage. Massage strokes relax your muscles *and* your psyche because being touched releases oxytocin; remember, that's the bonding hormone that makes you feel warm and fuzzy all over. It's the internal reason massages are so calming and soothing. The external one, of course, is how they unknot those tense, clenched muscles in your neck. You'll be instructed to book a massage on Day Two; maybe you should schedule two this week.

Profile Three: The Temporary Slump

Maybe you're going through a divorce, or you've remarried and become a blended family with stubborn stepkids, or you have a capricious, explosive boss . . . Whatever is going on, your confidence and self-esteem have plummeted and everyday irritants you'd normally blow off (cat hair on your best black pants, dead batteries in the remote) are getting to you at an alarming rate. Ideas to consider this week follow.

Take your mind off repeat. Sometimes problems swell into things that get out of control or look worse than they really are. And sometimes you just don't give yourself enough credit: You may actually be dealing with your daily stresses just fine, but in your head things feel frantic. Take a step back. Try to see yourself from someone else's eyes (anyone's eyes—your lover's, your gardener's, Big Bird's). You might see that you're actually doing better than you think. In that case, take that mind off repeat.

Crack Up to Crank Down

The health benefits of laughter are proven and plentiful, ranging from strengthening the immune system to reducing stress and food cravings and to increasing one's threshold for pain. Hormones, of course, are the reason. Health-promoting endorphins and neurotransmitters get released during a good laugh, and the number of antibody-producing cells and the effectiveness of certain immune cells also increases. An emerging therapeutic field known as humor therapy aims to help people heal more quickly with laughter. So take a load off and laugh!

Schedule a worry period. Okay, do you *relish* in worrying? Fine, worry away. But there's a catch: Devote two periods a day to it. Give your worries full attention for fifteen to twenty minutes. Wallow in them in all their soul-sucking glory. Then stop. When they rise up again, tell yourself that you'll address them during your next worry period. Now you're in control over *when* worries can worry you.

Laugh it off. No joke, there's something magical about laughter, even if it's forced. Laugh off some of the day's tensest moments. This is called *self-generated laughter* (versus cracking up at a comedian) and doing it regularly can make you more positive and optimistic. The reason's pretty basic: The more you laugh, the better you feel.

Let go of the past. Happy memories can be blissful, but obsessing over bad ones doesn't do any good. While learning from your mistakes can be productive, reliving them isn't. Focus on the present because the best thing you can do for yourself right now is exactly what you're doing with this vacation: destressing.

Profile Four: The Stress-Depressed, or a Woman on the Verge

The mortgage crisis hit and you lost your home. Your mom has developed dementia and no longer recognizes you. A single piece of bad news has sent your life into a tailspin from which you haven't been able to recover. You feel awful with good reason, and your body chemistry isn't helping. As the next chapter will begin to explain, those stress hormones that emerge when you're depressed undermine skin, weaken bones, set you up for diabetes, and fog your memory. If depression really gets a grip, it can actually shrink and damage a brain zone—the *hippocampus*—that, in turn, can prevent the shutoff of the entire stress response. More trouble, both on your inside and skinside. A few ideas to think about this week follow.

Take a decisive action. You're better off acting on stressful events than wishing really hard that they would just go away. But start simply. If you tackle one thing at a time, you can build a little momentum and see that things *can* get better.

Get more vitamin G. That's G for *green,* as in nature. Being outdoors among plants and other living things boosts your feelings of health and well-being. You don't need to live next to a lush forest. Find a park to take your daily walk in. Set up a favorite chair in front of the window with the best view. Buy a big philodendron (they're nearly impossible to kill) and place it in the room where you spend the most time.

Make big goals smaller. Persistently pursuing a big dream is great when you're getting somewhere. But if you're not, it's the stress pits. Repeatedly hitting dead ends can also make your levels of something called C-reactive protein—CRP, a marker of inflammation—rise. Since inflammation has been linked to depressive symptoms, stewing over going nowhere may add to your blues. Instead, let go of what's not working and replace it with smaller, newer, more reachable goals.

Take a ten-minute mind trip. Remember the last time you floated effortlessly in sun-warmed salt water? Or whooshed like an Olympic skier over fresh powder? You can go there any time you like, and reap the relaxing rewards, using your imagination. All it takes is a quiet spot, an easy chair or place to lie down, and ten or fifteen uninterrupted minutes. Eyes closed, bring to your mind an image of the place where you felt peaceful and happy. Now scan the scene from top to bottom, left to right and see little details—the way the sun reflected off the water or how the snow flew by. What did the breeze feel like on your cheeks? What sounds did you hear? How did the air smell? Relive as many things as you can. Feel the pure pleasure of being in that space and time. You'll soon feel as relaxed as if you'd actually been there.

Profile five: The Robot in a Rut

Something triggered a stress fest in your life and you responded by drinking too much, starting to smoke again, falling off the exercise wagon, and/or getting into a high-fat, sweets-laden, fast-food rut. In short, you slid into some unhealthy habits that you're having trouble breaking, even though you know they are just making things worse. Here's what to focus on during your program.

Tackle one habit at a time. This week, pick one habit you want to change, and be absolutely clear with yourself about why. If you smoke, fear of maybe getting lung cancer obviously isn't enough or you would have quit already. So think about the things that will definitely happen: the wrinkles and dryness that already show on your skin. The money you'll waste. The bad breath that makes people turn their heads aside when they give you a hug. Now write down all the reasons and read the list several times a day.

Stop telling yourself that you are bad because you have a bad habit. When you're stressed out, going back to an old habit that feels comforting is hard to resist (celebs don't seem able to do anything else). So, maybe you start smoking again or biting your nails or eating fries for dinner . . . which makes you feel bad . . . which is a sure route to reinforcing the habit. Instead, try to separate yourself from the habit—it's simply a behavior, not a definition of you—and you'll be better able to break it.

Hum. Literally. It boosts nitric oxide (NO), a nifty little body gas that in small doses has a stress-reducing effect. All of us produce the gas nitric oxide in our respiratory tract, notably in the nasal sinuses; in fact, every cell in the skin likely can produce NO, where it promotes wound healing, new collagen formation, and dilation of blood vessels in the dermis. Because nitric oxide can have a stress-reducing effect as well, encouraging its production is a good idea. A proven method? Classic humming, which oscillates the airflow in nasal passages to speed up the exchange of air between the sinuses and the nasal cavity.

Take baby steps. Small goals let you succeed every day, in tiny increments. And one success leads to another, and another.

Most of us fit into one or more of these five stress profiles. As women, we all get stuck in similar stress ruts at various times in our lives, and recognizing them for what they are makes it easier to combat them. Remember your profile and any additional items you highlighted, because these will be additional focal points in your program coming right up. If they are not specifically mentioned in the outlined protocol that follows, you'll want to add them for optimal results.

day one: simplify

- Out with the old, in with the new
- Establish a regular sleep schedule
- Beauty Bonus: Change bed linens

Step one is establishing a routine with sleep and your daily face-care habits. As Clarissa Riggins did, see if you can find an ideal time to say, "It's time to get ready for bed, which means winding down and washing up." And for many the code word here is *simplify*. You will simplify your beauty and bedtime routine.

When patients first come to me looking for help in boosting their skin health, I often ask them to bring in all their products so I can see what they use and where they may be going wrong. In most cases, they dump all their current supplies and start over. It's highly likely that you have been overtreating your skin with multiple products, many of which could be harsh and exacerbating—rather than relieving—irritation and inflammation that can lead to breakouts and other skin conditions. I also look to see that their products are noncomedogenic. If you see the term *oil-free* on a label, you're safe.

I recommend doing the same here and starting fresh. Just the thought of going out and buying a few items to replace your old ones has a psychological plus to it. And you don't need to go further than your local drugstore to pick up the following: a gentle cleanser you can use every day, and two good moisturizers, one with sunscreen for daytime use and another for nighttime use. Your daytime moisturizer can be extra special with antioxidants and your nightly cream can include an over-the-counter retinol product if you so choose. If you have acne, get yourself an antiacne formula as well, such as benzoyl peroxide, and while you're at it, pick up any kind of gentle exfoliator you want. It can be a salicylic acid toner or a fruit-enzyme-based formula with jojoba beads. (Refer to chapter 2 for more specifics on these, and the directions below.) The bottom line is this: Don't overdo it! Keep it simple. I see too many women who overtreat and overscrub their faces clean to the point that they defeat the purpose. Instead of boosting their natural glow and cell turnover, they end up causing irritation and inflammation. They trigger a cascade of localized stress-response events that lead to dryness and breakouts.

Directions: For optimal results, do the following:

1. Toss out all old skin and facial cleansing products.
2. Buy a gentle facial cleanser, a morning moisturizer with sunscreen, and a nighttime moisturizer.
    a. Apply facial cleanser in morning shower with bare hands.
    b. Apply daytime moisturizer while face is still damp; let it soak in before applying makeup.
    c. Apply nighttime moisturizer after cleansing face with hands again (you can use the same cleaning soap as your morning routine).
3. Have a trusted exfoliator on hand to use two to three times a week, or as needed.

Products that get my thumbs-up are listed below. By no means is this an exhaustive list; I just want to give you some examples to get started. Look for more ideas in the charts in chapter 10. Also, be advised that actual names of these products may change (or have changed since this writing).

Cleansers

Cetaphil Gentle Skin Cleanser

Purpose Gentle Cleansing Wash

Dove Sensitive Skin Foaming Facial Cleanser

Aveeno Ultra-Calming Foaming Cleanser

FOR ACNE-PRONE SKIN

Clinique's Acne Solutions Cleansing Foam

Clean & Clear Advantage Acne Cleanser

Topix Benzoyl Peroxide 5% Wash

Daytime Moisturizer

Eucerin Everyday Protection Face Lotion with SPF 30

Kinerase Cream SPF 30

Topix Replenix CF Anti-Photoaging Complex SPF 45

Neutrogena Healthy Defense SPF 30

Aveeno Continuous Protection Sunblock Lotion for the Face SPF 30

Nighttime Moisturizer

Aveeno Ultra-Calming Night Cream

Topix Replenix Cream

Cetaphil Moisturizing Lotion

Revale Skin Night Cream (contains coffeeberry)

WITH RETINOL

Philosophy Help Me Retinol Night Treatment

Topix Replenix Retinol Smoothing Serum 2X, 3X, and 10X (also contains green tea polyphenols)

Exfoliating Toners

Clinique's Clarifying Lotions (or try their 7 Day Scrub Cream Rinse Off Formula)

Kiehl's Ultra Facial Toner

Philosophy Microdelivery Peel Pads

Daily Microfoliant by Dermalogica

La Roche-Posay Effaclar Toner (If you are acne-prone, try La Roche-Posay Effaclar Toner Astringent Lotion.)

Plan to wash your face twice a day as I outlined in chapter 2—once in the morning and again just before bed. Go lighter on your makeup during the day, too (you don't have to buy a whole new set of makeup; stick with what you've got but don't overdo it). That takes care of your first order of business, and now we must find a way to get that free cosmetic medicine: sleep.

I aggressively treat sleep-deprived women regularly, many of them are amazed by how much restful sleep can make them look years younger. Scientists are finally beginning to figure out why sleep deprivation makes us so emotional. In studies they kept a group of healthy men and women up for thirty-five hours straight, then monitored their brains while they showed them a series of pictures that ranged from neutral to gory. At the sight of the nasty photos, their sleep-deprived brains lit up like a firestorm in an area of the brain—the *amygdala*—that is an emotional center, alerts the body during danger, and activates the fight-or-flight response (cortisol and adrenaline surges).

Normally, other parts of the brain weigh in and release chemicals that calm the amygdala. But when you are functioning on zero sleep, things go haywire: The amygdala stays in overdrive, which keeps the stress response going in an endless feedback loop. Bottom line: Sleep helps keep our emotions on an even keel. To help make sleep happen, follow this quick ritual every day of your program, and hopefully every day thereafter as well.

- **Four to six hours before bed:** Stop any caffeine (knock off even earlier if you're caffeine sensitive).
- **Two to three hours before:** Don't eat a full meal. Digesting food (especially a heavy meal) can keep you awake.
- **Sixty minutes before:** Turn off all electronics—yes, the television, too—and dim the lights. Even if you're in your jammies and not feeling wound up, light signals your brain to stay alert and mental stimulation (especially from video games, nightly news, *Sopranos* reruns) makes it harder to fall asleep.

- **Thirty minutes before:** Drink something you find soothing. It could be a cup of chamomile tea, warm milk, or a splash (*not* a glass) of brandy, red wine, or some other nightcap that relaxes you. Just limit alcohol intake because it can awaken you later. If you find it's a slippery slope, cut it out entirely and switch to herbal tea. Try a warm bath or light reading (no work!).

- **Five minutes before:** Make sure your bedroom is dark (or wear an eye mask), quiet (or get a white noise machine or ear plugs), slightly cool (or open the window), and free of distractions (clutter, pets, work piles). G'night . . .

Remember to go back to the ideas on pages 83–85 if you qualify as seriously sleep-deprived. You may not need a full eight or nine hours per night, but you probably have some sense of how much sleep you need from experience. You know, for example, that when you get exactly eight and a half hours, you feel great, and that anything below seven puts you on edge for days.

More people have a set time that they get up every morning due to the day's responsibilities (the time you need to get the kids up or get to work yourself), so it's more difficult to change that determined time. It's much more practical to set an exact bedtime for yourself and promise not to stay up past that time. Starting today, calculate back from your wake time the hours you think you need to feel refreshed and energetic tomorrow. If it's eight hours, which is what I suggest if you don't know, and you normally rise at six, then that means calling it a day at least by nine at night, which gives you a final hour before your ten o'clock bedtime to relax and unwind. It typically takes a person twenty to thirty minutes to fall asleep, so if you want to get even more precise, plan to be in bed with the lights out at least twenty minutes *prior* to

Sleep Three Years Off!

Logging eight hours of sleep per night can make your RealAge as much as three years younger. Sleep deprivation lowers circulation, which is why you lose facial color and look pale and washed out. You can't wake up glowing after only a few restless hours of Zs.

your actual bedtime. In our example, that would be 9:40 P.M. Forty minutes is plenty of time to ready yourself for bed and do something soothing.

Day One Tip. Sometimes we jump into self-help routines without much thought, go through the motions, then drift away after a few days. I don't want that happening to you. Right here on Day One, mentally get into it—spend at least fifteen uninterrupted minutes focusing on why you're doing this, all the good things you're going to get out of it, and what you want to accomplish in the next eight days. Then go for it. It's going to do great things for you!

Beauty Bonus. Change your sheets and pillowcases today; there's no sense in applying anything to your face at night if you are cozying up to bacteria. Make it a goal to change your sheets and pillowcases at least one a week. Wash in hot water.

day two: relax

- Daily skin care routine
- Maintain sleep schedule
- Book a massage, connect with friends, and/or have sex
- Establish daily breathing exercises
- Beauty Bonus: Safflower oil

If you started this program on Saturday, then today is Sunday and it's time to schedule at least two important beautifying to-dos: time with friends or a massage, and sex. And I want you to learn a few great breathing exercises that you can perform *daily*. If you have never taken the time to stop and practice a few deep belly breaths throughout your day, you are in for a treat. It's remarkable what a few simple breathing exercises can do to calm you, refocus your energy, and literally change your body chemistry so that it supports happiness from the inside out. A five-minute breathing exercise can help keep cortisol levels in check and psychologically prepare you for more battles that day. You'll find yourself taking things in stride rather than letting every little thing rattle you.

I'll get to those breathing exercises shortly; let's start with what could be your biggest challenge today: sex. I know that for many women, sex isn't something you can do at the drop of a hat. With many couples, especially those who lead very busy lives and who both work, it may require penciling in the occasion (to at least get your partner on the same playing field!). Let your partner know well in advance that you plan on sex today, whether it's afternoon sex or after the kids have gone to bed. If you don't have a partner right now, then pleasure yourself! Yes, *masturbate*. You can reap the same benefits even though you don't have a human participant (see "The Sex Connection" on page 98).

I also encourage you to make an effort today to connect with friends. You can do this by picking up the phone and calling someone you haven't spoken with in a long time. (Later in the week, you'll be having dinner with friends so maybe invite the ones you call to your Thursday night powwow.) Just don't call anyone you would place on your toxic list, or someone you know will do nothing but complain to you about everything terrible that's going on in her life and the world. You want to connect with someone who makes you laugh, and who can take a load off your stress level and help you put things into perspective.

Following are three great breathing exercises that I enjoy. Try them all, pick the one that feels best, and use it often—at least twice a day during your program. It helps to choose a time when you take a breathing time-out each day. By practicing your breathing exercises at the same time, say first thing in the morning and in the midafternoon when life's busyness seems to peak, you will reinforce a pattern so that this practice becomes routine.

To experiment with the exercises, sit in a chair with your back comfortably upright, feet on the floor, shoulders down, chest open, and hands resting in your lap. Let your abdomen expand on each inhale and contract with every exhalation. You may want to close your eyes and really focus on your breaths

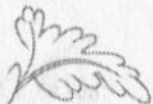

The Sex Connection It's real. Sex, especially in a loving, secure relationship (no fear, no anxiety, no "is he going to call me?" stuff going on!) is a bonus for our health and beauty. In addition to all the stress-reducing hormones that get released, giving us feelings of pleasure, elation, and no pain, regular sex is regular exercise and has similar benefits, including improved cholesterol levels and increased circulation. It also has been shown to boost immunity and reduce one's risk for heart disease.

One British researcher, Dr. David Weeks, a clinical neuropsychologist at Scotland's Royal Edinburgh Hospital, conducted a large-scale, long-term study and found that sex helps you look between four and seven years younger. Dr. Weeks attributes this to significant reductions in stress, greater contentment, and better sleep. What's more, he believes (and so do I) that an active sex life actually slows the aging process. The health-boosting benefits are not surprising when you think about what happens when you're in the act: Within a half hour your heart races, your breath gets deeper, and blood flow to your brain and other organs, skin included, increases.

The icing on the cake is that you can burn about as many calories having sex as you would doing weight training or walking at three miles per hour. Sex might even be as good as a sleeping pill: The relaxing chemicals released around the time of orgasm stick around for five minutes to an hour afterward, depending on the chemical, and that may explain why people too stressed out to go to sleep drift off more easily after sex.

The research has gotten wild in some regards. Researchers have found that mood-altering hormones in semen pass through the walls of the vagina and, within a few hours, are circulating in your bloodstream. Even if you're not in a long-term monogamous relationship that allows you to have condomless sex, you can still benefit from being intimate with your partner or even yourself due to all the other mood-enhancing effects that accompany sex. As long as you keep it safe (self-pleasuring definitely counts here), sex is great for health in general.

as you do this. Many of us breathe shallowly throughout the day without even realizing it. As we run around on autopilot, filled with mental tension, we tend to cut our breaths short, and even hold in our bellies and restrict the flow of oxygen. You will notice a difference once you pay attention to the movement of your diaphragm and the expansion of your chest. Let everything relax, including your stomach. As you inhale, you should feel your belly and ribs expanding, and then as you exhale, you'll feel them collapsing.

1. **Let it all out.** Take a deep breath through your nose and let it out easily through your mouth. At the end of the exhalation, silently repeat, "la-la-la-la-laaah," which effortlessly extends it, releasing more air from your lungs. Feel your abdomen inflate with the next inhale. Do five times.

2. **Take a pause.** Inhale and exhale through your nose, mentally counting, "in-two-three, out-two-three," and then "pause-two-three." During the pause, don't breathe in or out; just rest comfortably. Do five times. Over time, increase the count to four ("in-two-three-four, out-two-three-four"), then to five, until you reach a number that's comfortable to you.

3. **Hold it.** This technique can help you dial down a stressful reaction to upsetting news, and it help you fall asleep, too. It takes a little practice, but people who use it swear by it. It's a favorite of health guru Andrew Weil, MD, who calls it the "four:seven:eight breath."

- Place the tip of your tongue just behind your upper front teeth; let it rest there gently for the entire exercise.

- Exhale completely through your mouth, letting the air make a whooshing sound as it passes out.

- Close your mouth and inhale through your nose as you mentally count to four. Let the breath fill and expand your abdomen as you inhale, then hold your breath for a count of seven.

Exhale through your mouth with a whoosh to a count of eight. That's one complete four:seven:eight breath. Do four times.

Again, plan to perform at least one of these breathing exercises twice a day. On Day Seven I'll teach you how to meditate and you can see which form of relaxation you like best.

Day Two Tip. If you started the program on Saturday, then it's already time to protect yourself from the stress of the coming workweek by planning ahead. Think about doing your grocery shopping now, when you are not rushed. Make sure you pick up plenty of lean proteins (eggs, chicken, chickpeas, shrimp) and healthy snacks (berries galore, other fruits, dark chocolate, walnuts), so you won't be swayed when temptation rises. Flip to chapter 7 if you need tips to choosing well. If you have children, it may also be helpful to have a conversation with your husband or partner to split up more of the duties. For example, if you're the one who regularly cooks, cleans, and readies the house for nighttime, then maybe it's time for your partner to take on a little more this week on the home front. Get his support on seeing you through this program, especially during the workweek when life can move at lightning speed. If you have a small child who frequently needs attention in the middle of the night, let your husband be the caretaker. He may be grumpy at first, but he'll get his own reward later when you emerge from the program more vibrant, more beautiful, and definitely more sexy.

Beauty Bonus. Recall the benefits that safflower oil, which is high in moisturizing linoleic acid, can have on your driest skin spots. When you get out of the shower today, have some ready to slather on those trouble spots. You can, if you choose, use it on any dry body part, but stay below the neck. It's my favorite for dry lower legs, where flakiness can be especially persistent. The oil is pressed from the seeds of spiky yellow safflowers; in theory you could use olive oil, too, which is also high in linoleic acid, but you'd smell like a salad. Along with being odorless, safflower oil has the advantages of being colorless and cheap. If you are not sure about moisturizing with pure cooking oil (and the beauty industry sincerely hopes you aren't), you can find safflower oil in moisturizers, lip balms, and scrubs. Look for a product that lists it among the first three ingredients, which means it contains a high concentration of the oil. Otherwise, just pour some safflower oil into a pretty little squeeze bottle and add it to your toiletries. No one will ever guess you cook with it, too! And your legs will look amazing.

day three: go green

- Daily skin care routine
- Maintain sleep schedule
- Book a massage, connect with friends, and/or have sex (choose one you haven't done yet)
- Continue daily breathing exercises
- Get out in nature and take in your surroundings
- Beauty Bonus: Cleopatra milk bath

I'm crazy about tea, especially green tea. I go for black tea before noon, then switch to green tea (hot or iced) for the afternoon. Drinking green tea is one of the healthiest habits you can start. In fact, a 2006 European study, published in the *European Journal of Clinical Nutrition*, found that tea is a healthier choice than almost any beverage, including pure water, because tea not only rehydrates as well as water, but it also provides a rich supply of flavonoids (also called *polyphenols*), including catechins and their derivatives. One notable catechin called *epigallocatechin-3-gallate* (EGCG) is believed to be responsible for most of the antioxidant and anticancer properties linked to green tea. Catechins should be considered right alongside the better-known antioxidants, such as vitamins E and C, as potent free radical scavengers.

Most of the research showing the health benefits of green tea is based on the amount of green tea typically consumed in Asian countries—about three cups per day (which would provide 240–320 mg of polyphenols). As part of your Go Green day, I want you to make a big thermos of green tea at home and sip on it all day—hot at first, poured over ice later, if you like. Try doing this every day this week. In addition, make it a goal to get out in nature for at least twenty minutes today and each day during the remaining program to soak in some vitamin G. Nature can be extremely therapeutic. You're outside, where you can literally take in a breath of fresh air. It's true that the air is more toxic indoors than out, even if you live in a city like Los Angeles or New York. Indoor pollutants are silent and invisible. They come from your electronics, furniture, carpets, paints, heating and air-conditioning units. Getting outside is one of the best things you can do to lessen your exposure to pollutants and the very elements that trigger free radicals. And just taking a long walk in the comforts of your neighborhood or by work will suffice. I guarantee it will be rewarding in more ways than one.

Tea with a Twist

Add a squeeze of lemon to your tea and you'll up the number of catechins your body can absorb by 80 percent. Citrus boosts antioxidant absorption.

Here's one walk you might want to try. Step outside and leave your stresses—and your iPod—behind this time. Take in the details of your surroundings—the buzzing traffic or the birds, the curvature of plants and trees, the precise color of the sky and the shape of moving clouds. These are the details we rarely appreciate in daily living. You will find yourself becoming hyperaware and in the moment, and then I want you to think about what you are exceptionally thankful for in your life. It can be general or specific: your health, your family, your experiences at work, your life partner, your children, your last birthday party, and so on. Let your mind and memory run free. When you become very present like this, you start to think in a whole new light and connect in ways you never imagined. You also begin to get inspired, thinking more broadly rather than focusing on your own inner world and those trivial frustrations. This is a great way to beat down stress while at the same time appreciating where you are right now. It's especially helpful for those who fit the stress-depressed model. Also recall that one of my seven habits for healthy skin (number four, to be exact) entails focusing on the good things. When you are done with your walk, take five minutes to write down some of your revelations in a journal.

Day Three Tip. If something (or someone) starts to go crazy at home or work, immediately start a breathing exercise. Then either try to get outdoors for some vitamin G (and perspective) as soon as possible, or take one of the extra help steps for your stress profile type.

Beauty Bonus. If Cleopatra indulged in all the beauty treatments attributed to her, she wouldn't have had time to rule her empire, seduce Marc Antony, or learn Egyptian. But a girl's gotta bathe, so the one skin smoother she probably did rely on—milk baths—no doubt helped her bring Caesar and Marc to heel. Did Cleo know something we've forgotten? Actually, yes.

Milk is a super soother for chapping, windburn, sunburn, eczema, and other skin irritations. It contains proteins (whey and casein), fat, amino acids, lactic acid, and vitamins A and D, all of which calm dry, upset skin. Milk's lactic acid, in particular, weakens the glue that lets dead, ready-to-be-shed cells stick to the skin's surface, making it look dull and dry.

You can apply compresses dipped in cool whole milk for irritations like sunburn and eczema. Be sure to use whole milk; skim won't do because it doesn't contain fat, one of milk's most soothing components. If compresses aren't practical or you want a full-body effect, a milk bath will give you some relief. Try this tonight as part of your unwitching hour before bed: Add two to four cups to a warm (not hot) tub and soak for twenty minutes. You can use powdered whole milk, too. Sprinkle the amount of powder needed to make a quart of milk under the faucet as the water flows out. After your twenty-minute soak, give your body a gentle neck-to-toe scrubdown with a bath brush, loofah, or washcloth. This will slough off those dead cells, leaving skin smoother and softer. Apply moisturizer while your skin is still damp after you get out.

If you don't want to pour milk from your kitchen into the tub, you can purchase products that contain similar milk-based ingredients for the same effect. For instance, Fresh Milk Formula Bath Foam (www.sephora.com) contains milk as well as shea butter and glycerine. But if your skin is very irritated or totally winter-whipped, try the real thing. It should leave your whole body feeling creamy.

day four: eat clean

- Daily skin care routine
- Maintain sleep schedule
- Book a massage, connect with friends, and/or have sex (choose one you haven't done yet, or try the honey mask as I will explain)
- Continue daily breathing exercises
- Get out in nature and think about all the things for which you are grateful
- Avoid fast food, fried food, and anything processed
- Beauty Bonus: Moisturizing honey mask

While I'll make my case in chapter 7 for not harping too much about diet, it's important to know that the food-mood connection (and the digestive hormones related to hunger and metabolism) can be a factor in your levels of cortisol. Maintaining stable blood sugars will help you regulate your mood, which can then help you control your level of perceived stress. Stress is the most commonly reported trigger of binge eating, and research has shown that high cortisol levels correspond to both central body fat and food intake. High cortisol levels are also associated with increased insulin levels, which then throws blood chemistry off balance alongside your mood and motivation. Even after a stressful moment has passed, the increased cortisol levels in the body can be linked to an increased food intake. And we all know what that means: potential weight gain. When patients complain about their waistlines and inability to achieve an ideal weight, in addition to their other dermatological issues, I understand where they are coming from. It's natural for our self-image, self-esteem, and beauty concerns to be directly related to any problems with weight. How much we weigh accounts for much of our appearance.

That said, let's focus today on eating as cleanly as possible—no artificial or processed anything. Yes, that includes refined sugar, soda (both diet and regular), and processed meats and cheeses. If you are accustomed to eating processed and refined foods, this may be a challenge, but see if you can do this for at least one day, and then as much as you can for the remaining days of the program. It can take time to wean yourself off highly refined carbs, but tune in to how your body feels as you do your best to stick with the meal plan I've laid out for you. This meal plan will keep your blood sugars balanced so you won't feel either sickly, stuffed or insanely famished. If you choose not to follow today's plan to a T, that's okay. All I ask is that you focus on healthy, lean proteins and stress-fighting foods. Use chapter 7's guidelines for more ideas.

Breakfast

One to two eggs, any style (feel free to add herbs, salsa, and/or avocado)

One cup low-fat vanilla yogurt topped with lots of blueberries or raspberries (fresh or frozen)

One slice of whole grain toast

or

One to two eggs, any style

One slice low-fat cheese

One slice Canadian bacon (it's surprisingly lean)

One vitamin C–rich fruit (e.g., orange, grapefruit, papaya, strawberries)

Midmorning snack

A fistful of raw walnut halves or sliced bell peppers dipped in hummus

Lunch

An open-faced tuna sandwich on whole-grain bread with a slice of low-fat cheese melted on top

A big pile of veggies

An apple or pear

or

An open-faced turkey sandwich on whole-grain bread

A double helping of veggies drizzled with a little olive oil

Fruit of your choice

Afternoon

Superfood Snack Edamame *or* Smoothie (recipe follows); these snacks pack a punch of delicious nutrition, including skin-healthy antioxidants and omega-3s

SMOOTHIE:

1 cup water, plain soy milk, or low-fat or skim milk

1 cup fresh or frozen berries of your choice (try a medley of raspberries, blueberries, and blackberries)

2 tablespoons flaxseed meal or flax oil

ice and agave nectar to taste

Optional: 1 scoop vanilla or chocolate whey protein powder

Combine water or milk, berries, and flax in blender. Cover and blend until smooth. May also add ice to make a thicker concoction, and/or agave nectar for a sweeter taste (start by adding one tablespoon). For an added punch of nutrition (and a great source of essential amino acids), add one scoop vanilla or chocolate protein powder. Natural-food stores carry a wide variety of protein powders; just be sure not to buy meal-replacement powder. Another option is to visit a natural health food store's juice bar and choose a concoction. Just be sure to avoid the shakes made with added sugar, or ice cream!

Dinner

Grilled fish (e.g., salmon, sole, sea bass, or tilapia) or chicken

Three servings of veggies (asparagus, zucchini, Brussels sprouts, green beans, broccoli)

One cup brown rice or whole-wheat couscous

Sliced melon and berries

or

A meal-sized salad with romaine lettuce, grilled chicken, cucumbers, onions, olives, sunflower seeds, tomatoes, fat-free feta cheese, and a few raw nuts (of your choice), tossed with balsamic vinegar and olive oil

Dessert

A small portion of a favorite—say, one-fourth cup ice cream with fruit, one small piece of dark chocolate, two small cookies, or a thin slice of angel food cake. For a yummy sweet treat that's full of protein, not fat, whip a little low-fat ricotta cheese with a whisk until it's light and mousse-like, then stir in lots of frozen mixed berries. Add a drizzling of agave nectar (you'll find this in the sugar and baking aisle at the market; it's sweeter than honey but has a more liquid consistency and won't spike your blood sugar as severely as honey can). Or sprinkle on a packet Sugar In The Raw if you like, but taste test first; the juice from the berries should be quite sweet.

Day 4 Tip. Drink water or tea throughout the day; try to keep up with sipping from your thermos filled with green tea. You can always spice up regular water by drinking sparkling water and adding a splash of natural (no sugar added) cranberry juice, which is rich in antioxidants. Drop in a wedge of lemon, lime, cucumber, or melon for added flavor.

Beauty Bonus. While you've got food on your mind, use some on your skin externally and try this moisturizing honey mask (treat your skin after dessert). Honey is a natural humectant, meaning it draws free water from inner tissues to the surface layers of the skin. That subtle fluid shift creates a plumping effect that temporarily improves the appearance of wrinkles, which is a nice way to give yourself a glimpse of what is to come. It also soothes dry, sensitive, or irritated areas. In addition, honey is a natural antiseptic, and, thanks to all its antioxidants, an age fighter, too. The high concentration of sugars gives honey germ-killing power, which is why it's been used for thousands of years as a topical remedy to encourage wound healing. Its thick, sticky consistency also makes it a natural protective salve, sealing out infection and creating a moist healing environment within. You can even use it in a pinch if you develop blisters and don't have any salves like Neosporin around.

Here is a honey mask that can be your relaxation technique for the day.

- Mix two tablespoons honey with two teaspoons whole milk.
- Warm slightly in the microwave.
- Smooth the mixture onto the face and lie down for ten minutes (relaxing, plus it avoids sticky drips down your front).
- Rinse off with warm water.

If you prefer a more cosmetic form, store shelves are swarming with honey-enhanced beauty products such as BeeCeuticals Organics' Honey Thyme Hand and Body Lotion, which is made from unfiltered, organic, nonirradiated honey (www.healthfromthehive.com). It's made to be gentle enough to use even on psoriasis or eczema. And Benefit's Honey . . . Snap Out of It Scrub (www.benefitcosmetics.com) has honey, vitamin E, and crushed almonds. Leave it on for three minutes and you've got a soothing and smoothing honey-almond mask. As for the age-fighting effects, all types of honey contain antioxidants that appear to block skin-cell-damaging free radicals, though dark honeys, particularly the honeydew and buckwheat varieties (check health food stores), have more of them than paler clover honeys. While there's still a debate as to how effective antioxidants are when applied to the skin, I think they are helpful. Honey happens to be versatile as a topical and a treat. I'm all for swirling dark honey into your yogurt every morning. It's a simple way to nourish your skin from the inside.

day five: make a move

- Daily skin care routine
- Maintain sleep schedule
- Book a massage, connect with friends, and/or have sex (choose one you haven't done yet, or repeat one)
- Continue daily breathing exercises
- Get out in nature and think about all the things for which you are grateful
- Avoid fast food, fried food, and anything processed
- Get active: Schedule at least thirty minutes of exercise
- Beauty Bonus: Manicure/pedicure or mask

No matter how busy a life you lead, I believe you should find time to fit in a regular exercise routine. You should be engaging in a physical activity at least thirty minutes or more at least three days a week that gets your heart rate up and makes you breathe a little harder. It doesn't have to be overly strenuous and you don't have to start training for a marathon or Olympic event. Whether it's a structured class at a gym, power walking with friends in the morning, danc-

Cool Off to Sleep

The effects core body temperature has on whether we feel alert or ready to doze off also explains how a hot tub, sauna, warm bath, and even exercise during the day can aid us in falling asleep easily and achieving more slow-wave, deep sleep at night. After you warm up in one of these activities, your body will cool itself way down in the hours afterward and help you to fall sound asleep at night. Taking a hot soak or sauna is also a great way to relax and take the edge off a stressful day.

ing, or renting DVDs with the latest from fitness trainers, there are lots of options. Get creative and have fun with your activity. Don't make it a chore, and don't make yourself miserable by doing something you hate. Exercise should be enjoyable—an outlet for stress rather than a trigger. Also bear in mind that many forms of exercise can involve your family and friends, which can be very motivating and offer an added benefit, especially psychologically.

Make today the day to do at least one thing (maybe two) more active than yesterday, and see if you can accumulate thirty minutes to an hour total of time spent getting your heart rate up. It's totally up to you what you choose to do, and can be as easy as putting your favorite tunes on an iPod and hitting the neighborhood pavement for a fast-paced walk.

More Proof: Exercise *Reverses* Aging

It sounds too good to be true, but one of the most exciting areas of study currently underway is how exercise can literally reverse aging. Just last year, researchers showed that exercise can help partially reverse the aging process at the cellular level. A team of Canadian and American researchers looked at the effects of six months of strength training in volunteers aged sixty-five and older. They took small biopsies of thigh-muscle cells from the seniors before and after the six-month period, then compared them with muscle cells from twenty-six volunteers whose average age was twenty-two. The scientists expected to find evidence that the program improved the seniors' strength, which it did by 50 percent. But they never expected what else they witnessed: dramatic changes at the genetic level. The genetic fingerprint of those elderly volunteers who'd gone through the strength training program was reversed nearly to that of younger people. In other words, their genetic profile resembled that of a younger group.

How did they measure this change and difference? At the beginning of the six-month period, researchers found significant differences between the older and younger participants in the behavior of six hundred genes. These particular genes become either more or less active with age. By the end of the exercise phase, a third of those genes had changed, and upon closer observation researchers realized that the ones that changed were the genes involved in the functioning of mitochondria. Mitochondria are your cells' generators, where ATP gets created to process nutrients into energy. Another way to look at this is to say you're only as old as your genes act.

Day Five Tip. You've just hit the halfway mark. Give yourself something special. Block out an hour today—one full hour—to do anything you'd like. Veg in front of the television, go shopping for some new makeup at a department store where you can get some TLC, get a manicure and pedicure, get that massage you still haven't had yet—it doesn't matter. Just make sure it's fun and relaxing and don't let anything interrupt it. This is quality you time.

Beauty Bonus. If you choose to relax in front of the television or go shopping (see today's tip), then add one more beauty-related undertaking today, such as getting a manicure/pedicure, or applying a mask and letting it dry as you watch your favorite television show. Here's one to try that you can pick up at any major drugstore: Burt's Bees Pore Refining Mask.

day six: foster friendships

- Daily skin care routine
- Maintain sleep schedule
- Book a massage, connect with friends, and/or have sex (choose one you haven't done yet, or try a yoga class)
- Continue daily breathing exercises
- Get out in nature and think about all the things for which you are grateful
- Avoid fast food, fried food, and anything processed
- Continue exercise routine
- Plan a dinner with friends or family
- Beauty Bonus: PM prescription

It's amazing how therapeutic time with special friends and family members can be, especially when it's in person. All too often we push socializing to the weekend (or several weekends out) and forget to connect with those we love. On this sixth day, let's aim to do just that. In the previous days, I hope you have found time to connect with friends at least over the phone or via e-mail. Now it's time to take it to the next level and see these beloveds in person!

I'll leave it up to you as to what exactly you want to do tonight. If you love to cook, by all means invite your friends and/or family members over for a scrumptious meal. You can also ask each of them to bring something and do it pot-luck style if you'd like. But if cooking (and cleaning up) isn't your thing, then find a great restaurant that's convenient for everyone and make a reservation. The point here is to get the people who are meaningful in your life—who make you laugh, and who inspire you—to come together and share stories and life experiences. Of course, please don't plan to eat at a fast-food joint. Splurge and treat yourself to a favorite restaurant, or a new one in town you've been dying to try. Give yourself permission to enjoy a fantastic meal with even-more-fantastic people.

Day Six Tip. If you and your dinner mates live close to each other, you can invite them back to your place for dessert and an after-dinner drink or wine. If it's winter, light up the fire and gather 'round. If it's summertime or balmy where you live, sit outside and create an atmosphere with candles (and more vitamin G). Go for an early dinner, though, so you're not up past your bedtime.

Beauty Bonus. If you are a smoker, make this the day you decide to quit and start taking the steps by enlisting a buddy to hold you accountable. Granted, quitting smoking is easier said than done. You will want to share your intentions with your doctor and explore any therapies available to you that can help you make this change. How to become smoke free is beyond the scope of this book, but make today the day you consider this courageous step. Here's a great start: Go to www.realage.com where you'll find the Stop Smoking Center and the "You Can Quit Plan." It's loaded with information and tips to kicking the habit, including a way to find a quitting buddy. Being part of a community where individuals all share the same goal can be tremendously helpful in your success. I can't express in words how powerful losing the cigarettes in your life can be when reversing the signs of aging and revitalizing your looks (and let's not forget health from the inside out).

Cigs Suffocate Skin

Smoking breaks down collagen and can cut oxygen flow to the skin by as much as 30 percent, giving it a lifeless appearance. All of my patients who smoke look older than those of the same age who don't.

day seven: pamper yourself

- Daily skin care routine
- Maintain sleep schedule
- Book a massage, connect with friends, try a yoga class, and/or have sex (choose one you haven't done yet, or repeat)
- Continue daily breathing exercises
- Get out in nature and think about all the things for which you are grateful
- Avoid fast food, fried food, and anything processed
- Continue exercise routine
- Plan a dinner with friends or family for next week
- Learn to meditate
- Beauty Bonus: Rescue dry hands and lips

By now you may feel like you've been pampering yourself all week long. But have you really been following my advice? I know that the third recommendation in particular ("Schedule a massage, connect with friends, try a yoga class, and/or have sex") has the most potential to be neglected over and over again. Today is the day you make sure to fulfill that goal. And I want you to take it one step further by adding any of the following: manicure/pedicure (if you haven't done this yet), haircut/styling, spa treatment. This will be a Friday for those who started the program on the previous Saturday, so it's usually easier to fit these types of luxuries into the schedule. Go for a mud bath or seaweed wrap. Whatever looks fun, exotic, and most of all, relaxing!

In the hour prior to your bedtime tonight, try to meditate. Remember, meditation has been shown to be associated with structural changes in the brain that may slow down the aging-related atrophy. In other words, meditation not only helps you better cope with stress, but it may also help you keep your brain young and functioning optimally. Here's a simple way to try it: Sit in a quiet comfortable spot (a chair is fine; you don't have to be cross-legged on the floor). Choose a word to repeat to yourself, like the familiar *ommm*. Although it's meaningless, its resonant sound has been shown to be calming. Or simply murmur "breathe in" and "breathe out" to yourself, or count your breaths from one to ten, then repeat. Close your eyes and focus on your word or count. When thoughts intrude, gently bring your attention back to the word or count. Don't stress over whether you're doing it right and, if time's an issue, set a timer so you don't worry about it. Otherwise, simply keep going as long as you can without falling asleep. When you're ready, slowly open your eyes.

If you've already noted some of the additional techniques at the start of this chapter for the emotionally fraught, then you may have already tried a worry session. This is when you devote a small pocket of time, fifteen to twenty minutes, to thinking about your main woes and stresses. For some people, especially those who suffer from insomnia because they let their worries consume their minds and rob them of the relaxation they need to fall asleep, it helps to actually write down their worries in a journal. Having them confined to paper lessens their heaviness and perceived burden. You may also find that solution to some of these problems emerge, for which you can then create a solution list. For example, if completing your tax returns has been eating away at you for weeks now because the deadline is looming, stop thinking about it and simply write down "schedule tax appointment with CPA" or "take fifteen minutes to work on taxes this weekend." You'd be surprised by how therapeutic this exercise can be for making those worries subside or become less significant in the minds. No matter what stress profile you call yourself, I encourage you to try this exercise tonight. Start a worry journal; you can also use a section of the same journal you may have started at the beginning of the program.

Day Seven Tip. Whether or not you've been keeping a journal and listing your worries at bedtime, try this exercise tonight: Write down three great things that happened today. They don't have to be out of this world. They can be as simple as the fact you got eight hours of sleep the previous night and you felt energetic all day, or that you hit a big deadline at work, or learned how to use a new weight-bearing machine at the gym. Just three good things, simple as that.

Beauty Bonus. Recovering dry, chapped hands and lips to their normal, supple state is relatively easy. This is a good exercise you can recall when the dead of winter hits. For hands, get yourself a pair of moisture-retaining cotton gloves (any drug or beauty store will carry these) and slather on a body lotion or hand cream before slipping into the lightweight gloves overnight. If your hands are extremely dry, you can go for a heavier formula like Burt's Bees Hand Salve, which contains botanical oils, herbs, and beeswax in a superrich, thick paste. Other brands I like include Cutemol or Triple Cream by Summers Labs.

To tame those flaming lips, get religious about applying your favorite lip balm or gloss throughout your day, one with sunscreen. Just be sure to skip the kind that contains phenol, like Blistex. Every time you think about licking your lips (or perhaps have just done so) get out the balm. Don't forget to apply a balm to your lips at night, too. That one doesn't have to contain sunscreen. Solid choices: Kiehl's Lip Balm #1 or plain old Vaseline. Kiehl's also makes a line of lip balms and glosses with sunscreen.

Nail Care 101

Nails can be windows to your overall health. Variations in texture and color can signal underlying medical problems, but you don't have to have any medical problems to have a problem keeping nails hardy. Some tips:

- Keep nails clean and dry. Wear cotton-lined rubber gloves when washing dishes. Repeated soaking and drying can dry your nail beds.

- Apply moisturizer to your nails and cuticles every day (this is especially helpful after every hand wash to lock in moisture). While any body lotion will do, creams with urea or phospholipids can help prevent cracking.
- Get plenty of biotin, a B vitamin known to promote healthy nails. Eat cauliflower, walnuts, and egg yolks to help increase the amount of biotin in your diet.
- Keep them polished, even if it's just clear nail polish. This can help protect brittle nails from splitting.
- Avoid nail polish that contain toluene and formaldehyde (can cause drying and contact sensitivity); avoid nail polish remover with acetone (too drying).
- Keep nails short so they stay out of harm's way. Don't cut the bottom cuticle because it's the barrier that keeps fungus, yeast, and bacteria out.
- Don't file to a point. File your nails in one direction and round the tip slightly.
- Bring your own instruments if you get frequent manicures. Be sure your manicurist doesn't beat up your cuticles too much; pushing your cuticles back can cause damage to the nail bed that leads to splits.
- The obvious advice: Avoid biting or picking your nails.

day eight: sleep-in beauty

- Daily skin care routine
- Maintain sleep schedule
- Book a massage, manicure, pedicure, spa treatment, hair appointment, connect with friends, try a yoga class, and/or have sex (choose one you haven't done yet, or repeat)
- Continue daily breathing exercises
- Get out in nature and think about all the things for which you are grateful
- Avoid fast food, fried food, and anything processed
- Continue exercise routine
- Meditate before bedtime
- Sleep in or try napping
- Beauty Bonus: Exfoliate

Assuming you have no early obligations today, I give you the free pass to sleep in as long as you like. Or if you are not the type to sleep in (either you just can't or don't like sleeping in), then try napping later in the day. The ideal time to nap is about eight hours after you awaken. This is when the body naturally takes a little dip in temperature as part of your normal biological rhythm (hence the afternoon lull for most—it's more a factor of your circadian rhythm than your lunch). A human's natural sleep pattern is *biphasic,* so twice during a twenty-four-hour period we all experience a drop in core body temperature that invites sleep. From a cultural perspective, this is probably why siestas came to be. Naps can provide a wealth of rewards that go beyond just making you feel better and able to tackle the rest of your day. Naps have been shown scientifically to benefit almost every aspect of human wellness, from the physical rewards of lowering your risk for heart disease and repairing cells to the more obvious ones of lifting your mood and stamina, knocking down stress, and making you more productive. Because naps can improve heart functioning, support hormonal maintenance, and encourage cell repair, they can help you live longer, stay more active, and look younger. Keys to napping:

- Set aside thirty minutes total—ten minutes to fall asleep and twenty minutes for the actual nap. Use an alarm.
- Take off your shoes, and get comfortable; try to nap in a reclined position on a couch or in your car (but be safe); avoid direct sunlight.
- Avoid napping past three in the afternoon. If you nap too late in the day, you can disrupt your nighttime sleep.

Napping isn't for everyone so see how it works for you. I also recommend using this evening to plan time with your significant other or a best friend. Get a babysitter if you need to, see a movie you've been dying to see, or have a nice, quiet meal at a place where you can share stories from the week.

Day 8 Tip. Keep the momentum going, and enlist your significant other or friend for help. Ask for input about how you look. Talk about the changes you've made and the things you want to keep doing to reduce stress in your life. Try to explain how you feel. Not only is sharing your success fun but enlisting a cheerleader will help you keep going. So when the day comes, and it will, when the kids are driving you mad, or you're ready to run over your boss, or your mother decides you've never fully appreciated what it took to bring you into the world, your cheerleader will help you laugh it off. For an added challenge, ask your trustworthy friend to call out your worst characteristic. Why do this? It's hard to look at ourselves in an unbiased manner. Your defense mechanisms kick in. However, this kind of evaluation will give you a new self-perspective that helps you to evolve and attract more people to you.

Beauty Bonus. Exfoliation can be done in a variety of ways. If you use an exfoliating toner in your daily routine (which is not necessary every day for most people), then this beauty bonus needn't apply to you. But if you have not exfoliated at all this week, now is the time to do so. Exactly which kind of exfoliating formula you want to you use is up to you (see chapter 2 or page 93 for specifics). If you scheduled a spa treatment today, then you can certainly take care of your exfoliation there.

day nine: reflect

- Daily skin care routine
- Maintain sleep schedule
- Book a massage, manicure, pedicure, spa treatment, hair appointment, connect with friends, try a yoga class, and/or have sex (choose one you haven't done yet, or repeat)
- Continue daily breathing exercises
- Get out in nature and think about all the things for which you are grateful
- Avoid fast food, fried food, and anything processed
- Continue exercise routine
- Meditate before bedtime
- Sleep in or try napping (hey, it's Sunday, isn't it?)
- Reflect on your week
- Beauty Bonus: Back to basics

Start thinking ahead. What is tomorrow going to look like? How can you make sure you keep up the good habits you're developing?

Feel free to add and subtract things that worked especially well for you during the last week, or didn't. Again, the point is to find what works for you, and that's going to be as individual as you, and your life, are.

You should be feeling really good about yourself. You are forming new habits that can change you for forever. And you've gotten into the groove of putting yourself first, which is important to learn because it isn't that easy for many of us to do (moms especially).

Over this ninth day you are going to seal the deal. Start by reflecting on what's gone well. Do you feel physically and emotionally better than you did last weekend? What helped most? Taking more vitamin G? Turning off all those electronic screens? Taking fifteen minutes sometimes to do *nothing*? Having more sex? Take note.

Now, consider a different kind of reflection: Look in the mirror. Really look. Of course I realize you've been watching for changes all along—and seeing some. But by Sunday afternoon on the second weekend, if you've followed the plan, I *know* you look not just younger but also happier and healthier and, okay, this is a little odd, but more *whole*. There's not just less stress in the mirror, there's more *you* there. You're back. Stay here!

Day 9 Tip. Pick the stress buster that you've liked doing best—meditating, four:seven:eight breathing, sex, having a worry session, whatever—and do it twice today. (Yes, you can have sex more than once a day! And your partner will love it, too.)

Beauty Bonus. Get back to basics today by doing nothing but your everyday skin care routine without added frills or total body treatments. Let your morning and nighttime routines take no longer than three minutes (gentle cleansing, moisturizing, and sunscreen in the morning; gentle cleansing, maybe gentle exfoliation, and nighttime creams/serums for the PM treatment). Of course, I'll give you an extra minute or two to take care of any special issues like acne with spot treatments or smoothing on a prescribed retinoid. Whatever you do, make today all about simplicity.

a beautiful day

Want to see what an ideal schedule looks like for someone who remains focused on the quality of her day—and looks? Here's a sketch of one beautiful day. Ask yourself how close can you come to this on a regular basis.

7:00	Wake up and do some deep breathing exercises (thinking positively about the day)
7:10	Shower and wash face and body with simple routine
7:30	Eat a lean, high-protein breakfast; prepare your thermos of green tea
10:30	Take a ten-minute stress break. Try doing something relaxing such as engaging in light conversation with a friend, or shopping online. Schedule a massage and manicure for the following day after work.
12:30	Eat a lean, clean lunch, followed by a short walk outside (vitamin G)
2:00	Take the other twenty minutes from your lunch hour and sneak in a twenty-minute nap
4:00	Do five minutes of deep breathing, then eat an apple
5:30	Hit the gym for a power yoga or aerobics class
7:00	Eat a protein-rich, relaxing dinner
9:30	Stop working, cleaning, or doing anything too stimulating; begin to wind down; consider a meditation session

10:00 Prepare for bed by washing up and winding down; have a light snack if necessary; write down in your journal a few things on your mind, and then three great things that happened today

10:30 Snuggle or cuddle with your partner. If it leads to sex, great. If you're alone, consider pleasuring yourself.

11:00 Lights out!

This is just one way to look at it. Someone might prefer exercise in the morning or at lunchtime. Another person may be an early riser, getting up at five and hitting the sack by nine. There are no hard and fast rules on how to plan the day. This is simply to show you how you can sneak in stress-reducing techniques and address your personal needs all day long. And you don't have to book a flight to Hawaii to do this! The whole point of the program is to show you how to achieve, and maintain, a lower stress level and a higher beauty state without having to resort to drastic measures.

Success and Sticking to It

It's time. Go ahead. Look in the mirror. Have the bags beneath your eyes lightened up? Do you look rested and energetic? How much younger do you look? Take the SkinAge test again.

Write down what you're happy with, where the biggest improvements are, and what you think can get even better if you stick with the program. And you can and should! Yes, this is a quick fix but it's also the first step toward a much happier, healthier way of living.

For the real proof as to why all my ideas in this program should translate to a more beautiful you, turn to the next chapter and start learning the ins and outs to stress aging. The knowledge you gain will affirm why you are practicing these habits that are the foundation of the program.

Record your results right here:

Top Five Ways I Look Better	*Top Five Things I Want to Continue Doing*

Q: My eyes look tired—a lot. Even though I'm following the program well, I still wake up with big, swollen eyes. Any quick fix I can use in the morning?

A: Eyes can look swollen from allergies, too much partying, too much computer time, too little sleep, or loose under-eye skin caused by heredity or aging. If you've been following the program, it may take longer to see the results, so be patient. But you may also have some hereditary issues that make it more challenging. Whatever the cause, here are three ways to deflate under-eye baggage fast.

- **Remember the power of the cucumber.** Veggies contain a combo of mild natural acids that reduce water retention. Some beauty pros say cucumbers work best when they're cold, which makes sense: Because cucumbers are 90 percent water, chilled slices are like delicate, little ice packs.
- **Reach for the peas.** Any bag of frozen food will do, but frozen baby peas have a way of fitting into the nooks and crannies around your eyes. Put a soft cloth around the plastic package to protect your skin from the frigid surface, then chill out for five to fifteen minutes while the cold shrinks the swelling. No peas? Rest a spoon in a glass of ice water for about thirty seconds, until it's really cold. Nestle the curved back of the spoon into the hollow of your eye, gently rolling it around,

for another thirty seconds; then rechill it and do the other eye. On a really bad morning, repeat. The cold will bring the puffy swelling down in a flash. Your whole body will feel a little more awake, and you'll feel ready to begin your day.

- **Make a milk bath.** Milk (whole, not skim) is a natural soother if eyes are irritated as well as puffy. Other ingredients in milk that calm swollen skin include protein, amino acids, lactic acid, and vitamins A and D. Pour milk into a bowl of ice so it gets really cold, saturate a clean washcloth, and apply to eyes for up to fifteen minutes. Soak and reapply when the cloth loses its cool.

P.S. If puffy eyes are a chronic problem, eye-shaped packs filled with gel that freezes are a worthwhile investment . . . and they don't drip.

5

how stress gets under your skin

Understanding the Mind-Beauty Connection

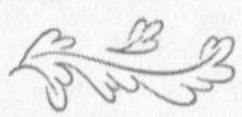

I had my first insight into this fascinating mind-beauty connection when I was just nine years old. My mom had been hospitalized for depression and, when we went to visit her, her appearance shocked me. She'd suddenly gotten *old.* She had dark circles under her eyes, gray and sagging skin. Not the mom I had ever known. Even her hair was dull. Yet she was just thirty-three—a woman in her prime! Clearly, depression had aged her prematurely. But equally amazing was what happened next. When the depression lifted, so did the years. She had responded well to treatment and therapy, arriving home looking like my mom again. She had reclaimed her youthful looks and vitality.

It doesn't take a case of full-blown depression to add years to your physical body. How many women do you know who walk around in a state of chronic exhaustion and stress? Or who reel from one emotionally fraught problem to another—with their marriage, weight, job, finances, kids, whatever on their mind—and have almost forgotten how to smile? While men can certainly fall into this same trap, I find that as women we are especially prone to the misgivings of overscheduled and overcommitted lives, particularly given the roles we accept in society (mom, wife, daughter, caretaker, homemaker, dog walker, bookkeeper, friend, mentor, employee or business owner, and so on).

Not surprisingly, women report feeling the effects of stress on their physical health more than men do. We rob from our precious sleep time to pay the bills, keep everyone else happy at home and work, and check off the to-do list. This also sets us up for falling into many unhealthy habits such as avoiding exercise, drinking too much alcohol, losing sight of what a healthy meal is, and resorting to lots of processed foods that will do exactly what we don't want to happen: pack on weight and age prematurely.

For the most part, though, we manage to keep all the balls in the air. But you've probably noticed that when the juggling act goes on for too long or when life throws you a curveball—your mom gets sick, or your partner loses his job, or the car *and* the hot-water heater call it quits on the same day—your looks take a dive. Whether it's dark circles, pallid patches, a giant pimple, or what looks like a whole new set of crow's feet, it's the final insult.

That's a classic sign of stress aging. It's what happens when an overload of life adds years to your looks. It can age your face far more rapidly than the passage of time. Here's the shocker: *Stress can age you three to six years or more.* And it's a familiar, vicious cycle: Stress affects your beauty, and when you're not happy with your appearance, you're not happy in general and you can't cope with stress so easily. Which then comes back to take a bite out of your beauty again and again. Oh, and don't for a minute think that this is a female thing, even though I'm focusing on us women here. Think of how Bill Clinton or George W. Bush looked before they entered the Oval Office compared with their appearances near the end of their terms. The presidency gave them power, prestige, and . . . white hair, deep creases, blotchy complexions, and extra pounds.

Now that you've got your list of to-dos and

Octogenarians on the Rise

Baby girls born in 2004 can expect to live to the ripe age of eighty, a new record. So, it's more important than ever to feel happy in your own skin. Consider it a birthright not only to want to live longer, but also to remain and look radiantly healthy.

have set a program in motion, it's time to get a behind-the-scenes look at why this program works. I think virtually everyone agrees by now that stress is, for the most part, unhealthy, and that perpetual, long-term stress can make you sick, but it's not commonly understood just how this is true from both a biological and psychological standpoint. The evidence might surprise you.

anatomy of stress

Stress is a wily adversary. It has a lot of sneaky ways to get under your skin and inflict damage. Millennia ago, when threats were more clear-cut, human beings relied on the famous fight-or-flight response to prime our bodies for battle or to vanish in a flash whenever a saber-toothed tiger stalked us for lunch.

But Darwin is dead, and for the last several hundred years, humans have been taken out of the survival-of-the-fittest Darwinian jungle. These days, stress is most likely to come at us from bumper-to-bumper commutes, overbearing bosses, overbooked babysitters, tainted lettuce, concerns about global warming . . . the list of modern life's aggravators and dangers is so endless, it could wrap around the planet. And, unlike a confrontation with one of those big-fanged cats—it pounces, you lose, end of story—modern stresses can often be relentless, chronic, and cumulative.

Stress physiology has come a long way in the last century, especially in the last fifty years, thanks to major advances in medicine and public health. Think about it: Your great-great grandparents probably worried about diseases like scarlet fever, polio, malaria, influenza, and perhaps the thought about giving birth. Today we are more likely to die old and worn out;

Stress Fracture

When the demands placed on us exceed our perceived ability to cope, we experience *stress*. Stress is also defined as the thoughts, feelings, behaviors, and physiological changes that happen as a result of our response to those demands and perceptions. A whopping 82 percent of women say they have had at least one physical stress symptom in the last month such as a relentless headache, an upset stomach, or tightness in the chest.

we succumb to age-related diseases that slowly build up over a lifetime and present themselves . . . eventually. They include heart disease, cerebrovascular disease, and cancer. I love how Robert M. Sapolsky explains this in his book *Why Zebras Don't Get Ulcers:* "While none of these diseases is particularly pleasant, they certainly mark a big improvement over succumbing at age twenty after a week of sepsis or dengue fever." He then goes on to say that coinciding with this relatively recent shift in the patterns of disease have come changes in how we perceive the progression and the process of disease.

Stressless Fact

As the irony of life would have it, apparently stress is something we handle better with age. All of us react differently to stress and stressful events but, on average, it seems we become better equipped to handle stress the older we get. According to the National Study of Health & Well Being done by the University of Wisconsin-Madison Institute on Aging, older men and women (ages sixty to seventy-five) reported fewer daily stressors than their younger counterparts. And compared to people ages twenty-five to fifty-nine, older adults say their stress is not nearly as disruptive and unpleasant.

We now acknowledge and have been amassing the scientific proof of the delicate yet complex intertwining of our biology and our psychology—the untold ways in which our personalities, emotions, feelings, and thoughts both reflect and affect what's going on inside our bodies. There are lots of two-way streets here: Life has an impact on your body physically, and your body physically has a say in determining how well you feel and live, and whether or not you'd call yourself a happy person. Intangibles like emotional distress, personality traits, psychological characteristics, and even socioeconomic factors can all influence bodily processes including real, physical aspects to us such as our hearts, minds, nerves, and fat cells. It's an exciting time in medicine, when we are just beginning to understand how these intangibles can, as Sapolsky so eloquently explains, determine whether or not cholesterol sticks to your arteries, whether your pancreas stops producing insulin, thus giving you type-1 diabetes, or your cells stop responding to insulin, thus giving you type-2 diabetes, and whether or not your brain's neurons could survive a few minutes without oxygen if your heart stopped beating.

The paradox, of course, is that stress isn't always a bad guy. The pressure of competition or of meeting a deadline can raise your heart rate, alert your senses, and concentrate every cell in your body on acing a tennis match or perfecting a presentation. This stress-is-your-enemy-*and*-your-buddy conundrum has an enormous amount to do with hormones.

The Physiology of Stress in a Nutshell

When we think about hormones, those such as testosterone and estrogen likely first come to mind, but there's so much more to our endocrine system than the sex hormones that command our reproductive cycle. Every second of every day you have dozens of hormones acting in your body to get certain physiologic functions accomplished. These include reactions taking place in the skin, too.

Physiologically speaking, hormones control much of what we feel, be it tired, hungry, horny, hot, or cold. They control the rates of certain chemical reactions, assist in transporting substances through membranes, and help regulate water balance, electrolyte balance, and blood pressure. They manage development, growth, reproduction, and behavior. Put simply, hormones are the body's little messengers, which get produced in one part of the body, such as the thyroid, adrenal, or pituitary gland, pass into the bloodstream or other body fluid, and go to distant organs and tissues where they influence and change structures and functions. They are like traffic signals, telling our body what to do and when so it can run smoothly and efficiently. Hormones are as much a part of our reproductive system as they are a part of our urinary, respiratory, cardiovascular, nervous, muscular, skeletal, immune, and digestive systems.

When your hormones are not balanced or operating effectively, you will notice it. They can run amok in response to stressful periods or as a result of your age and condition (think puberty, pregnancy, menopause, etc.); they also can become imbalanced under the influence of a disease or an invading pathogen that changes the climate of your body. Because hormones hold this magic wand in us, if the wand isn't working properly we can experience a cascade of health problems, from a sluggish metabolism to infertility, diabetes, insatiable cravings, and so on. Skin conditions like acne, psoriasis, eczema, and rosacea can also be part of this mix. Then, suddenly, one problem becomes two, three, and four subsequent problems, such as unexplained weight gain, chronic pain, irritability, hair loss, fatigue, a loss of libido, and a general sense that something is not right. We feel tired and weak, unable to participate in life to its fullest.

Let's look at a few important hormones in particular that relate directly to stress and how our bodies cope with it. You've already heard many of these in the previous chapters, but here I'll help you gain a clearer understanding of how they can have a direct impact on your appearance.

Driving Under the Influence

Your body is constantly under the mercy of chemical substances, called *hormones*, that have a commanding role in many bodily functions. They can change your metabolism (make it faster or slower), affect your fertility, dictate your complexion and skin health, and even have a say in how well you can cope with stressful events. The chief hormones that come into play with regard to stress include adrenaline and cortisol.

The HPA Axis

When stress first attacks—whether the threat is emotional (bad news about a best friend) or physical (getting trapped in a blizzard)—the brain's first reaction is to signal to the adrenal glands to release *epinephrine*, better known as *adrenaline*. Among its many jobs are increasing heart speed and rushing blood to the big power muscles, just in case you have to move fast.

Adrenaline commandeers some of that blood from the skin and face, by the way, which makes you look washed out, which is where the phrase "white with fear" comes from. If whatever caused your heart to race passes, the adrenaline flow abates, your pulse assumes its usual pace, your palms dry, your color returns, and life as your body knows it goes back to normal.

But if your stress response gets kicked up another notch, a whole SWAT team of stress hormones kicks in to ready your body systems for action. Here's the 1-2-3 of what happens when a crisis hits:

1. The region of the brain called the hypothalamus releases a stress coordinator called corticotropin-releasing hormone (CRH).

2. CRH rushes over to the pituitary, a pea-sized gland at the base of the brain, and tells it to release adrenocorticotropic hormone (ACTH) into the bloodstream.

3. Fast-talking ACTH tells the adrenals (yep, they're called into action again) to release a major stress hormone, cortisol.

This sequence of events is known in scientific circles as the hypothalamic-pituitary-adrenal axis, or HPA axis. It is your body's main stress-response system. Think of it as old-fashioned messengering in a kingdom in the midst of war—a way of getting the word out to the body that it's time to mobilize the troops and prepare for battle.

And as you'll soon find out, your skin has a similar such system all on its own. To wit: The skin is the queen's twin, and a mistress in her own kingdom.

Cortisol, the hormone that has been echoing through these pages since the start of this book, actually breaks down tissue, including skin. It also can wreak havoc on numerous bodily functions. As your body's chief, and powerful, stress hormone, it tells your body to do three things: increase your appetite; stock up on more fat; and break down materials that can be used for quick forms of energy, including muscle. It sounds opposite to what you'd like to have happen, but that's how your body naturally responds to stress. It automatically goes into a protectionist mode. You see, cortisol is your primary *catabolic* hormone, meaning it halts growth and reduces cellular synthesis (as opposed to increasing cell production and metabolism), causes

Stressful Fact

The average American has about fifty brief stress attacks a day. The troops don't get much sleep.

muscles to break down, and assembles fat. It thinks the body won't see food again for a while or that it will need an ample supply of fuel to get through a rough patch. Clearly, one of the goals of this program is to control your cortisol levels naturally through modifications in your lifestyle, including diet, exercise, and relaxation techniques. And when you do manage your cortisol levels well, you can experience numerous benefits, from better skin to better weight control.

Cortisol's Clockwork

Cortisol levels are highest early in the morning and during periods of high stress, and lowest in early stages of deep sleep. Yet another reason to get quality shut-eye. You give your body the ultimate break from the madness.

That said, let me add that you wouldn't be alive without cortisol: It's the hormone that helps immune cells go after infectious invaders, then signals all clear to the brain when the battle is won. It also builds up energy reserves, warehousing calories that might be needed to fuel muscles for action, and does many other good deeds. You just want to be sure that it's around when you need it, and that it's gone when you don't. Because too much cortisol spells t-r-o-u-b-l-e.

If the crisis is prolonged, for instance, or another pops up and then another, cortisol and other stress hormones just keep pouring into your system. That's *chronic* stress and your body doesn't like to be in this unending, high-wire state. While the cortisol is there to pump you up, you probably don't need to lift cars or jump off a fire escape. Yet it keeps on flowing, taxing every system and organ in your body, including your skin. It can also disrupt the formation of *new* collagen, and sluggish collagen production makes skin thinner and weaker. Blood vessels become more fragile. It's skin aging in a nutshell: As the skin loses its capacity to hold on to moisture and becomes less resilient, permanent lines become more visible on the surface. New skin cells don't form as quickly, and cell turnover may eventually slow by half. Without a good blood supply, oil glands slack off and skin becomes dryer still.

The Collagen-Cortisol Connection

Let's back up a minute and explore this all-important tissue called *collagen,* which has such a defining role in our looks. It's our body's most abundant protein. About one-third of all proteins in our body is collagen, and about 90 percent of skin tissues owe their structure to collagen. It's continually undergoing a process of breakdown and repair, a cycle called *turnover,* to ensure our body remains in peak health. Because the skin is made up of so much collagen, it's more adept at handling stress and repairing cells after damage. You know this if you have ever slightly burned your arm while cooking. A few days later, your skin looks likes it's on its way back to normal. If you've ever felt sore after a hard workout or a day of skiing, you know that your body will feel normal again in a few days. What happens is the damaged muscle tissues (and tendons and ligaments, all rich in collagen) get repaired relatively quickly. Your body's turnover factory will remove damaged tissue and replenish it with new, stronger tissue. What happens when we age, however, is that this turnover process slows, and we become more vulnerable to tissue damage. We are likely living with decades of accumulated stress and less-than-perfect repair along the way.

In addition to cortisol's impact on collagen breakdown, other factors can contribute to skin damage. Chief among those factors are three things: glycation, oxidation, and inflammation. Here's the rundown:

Glycation. This is a natural process in which the sugar in your bloodstream attaches to proteins, forming harmful new molecules called *advanced glycation end products* (ironically, AGEs for short). The most vulnerable proteins are collagen and elastin, the fibers that you know by now keep skin firm and elastic. Researchers are currently trying to figure out just how this process factors into the age equation; it's not necessarily accurate to say "sugar causes wrinkles," because there are some complex biological pathways happening that involve more than sugar alone. Too much glycation may affect what type of collagen you can build, which is a huge factor in determining how resistant your skin will be to wrinkling. The damaging effects sugar can have on your looks is clearly evident in diabetics who have a hard time controlling their blood-sugar levels. Diabetics often show the signs of premature aging because they can go for years with undetected high blood sugar, causing them to physically age quicker.

Oxidation. One term you're likely already familiar with explains oxidation, and that term is *free radicals*. These are the loose cannons, highly reactive forms of oxygen to be exact, that can damage cell membranes and other cellular structures in the body, but especially in the skin. Free radicals attack us from a variety of sources, both internal as an outcome to normal metabolism and respiration, as well as from external sources like pollution and UV rays. In this program we are controlling exposure to free radicals and taking the steps necessary to address the damage that may have already done. Yes, you can control free-radical damage through specific protocols that entail treatments to the skin, as well as nourishment from the inside.

Inflammation. Like cortisol, inflammation has both pros and cons, and we very much need this protective mechanism. Inflammation is our bodies' natural response to injury or illness, helping us to survive. It's what helps kill an invading bacteria or virus, for instance. In today's world, we are at the mercy of too much inflammation all around. An overreactive inflammatory response is what triggers allergies and some autoimmune diseases, like arthritis. The response can also be misdirected, causing more skin damage and pain instead of less. To make matters worse, the presence of excessive free radicals, AGEs, and cortisol combined is like coarse salt in the wounds, leading to so-called hyperinflammation. No one in a hyperinflamed state will look good.

The solution: Get control of all these factors in the beauty equation. And that's one of the main goals of this program. These metabolic factors—all of which are linked to acne, wrinkles, discoloration, sagging, and the very process of not only skin aging but aging itself—can be brought under your control easily with a few simple strategies.

Why Chronic Stress Is So Chronically Bad

Chronic, unrelenting stress—the kind that modern life is too full of—changes your brain and body in all sorts of ways. Memory slips. Blood pressure rises. You gain fat around your belly, the unhealthiest place to put on pounds. This is called *visceral fat* because it's deeply embedded around your vital organs, thus increasing your risk for heart disease, cancer, and other illnesses. Your immune system takes a hit and you become more susceptible to infections. (Which explains why you're more likely to get a cold when you are overworked or overwrought.) Wound healing slows by as much as 40 percent, oil glands go into overdrive, and inflammation takes off. Plus, free radicals proliferate and run wild, subtly damaging skin and eventually drying it out, creating wrinkles and turning softness to sag.

What's more, some elements within the skin, including the hair follicles, are supersensitive to stress hormones. This may explain why some people lose their hair or grow it in the wrong places after a serious bout of emotional stress as hormones send the wrong message or no message at all. (More on this shortly.) No, stress has nothing to do with the growing shag on your husband's back—that's caused by different hormones!

Unfortunately, the ability to turn off the stress response, and return cortisol levels to normal, appears to decline with age. And, as these negative factors persist, your antioxidant defense mechanism takes a hit, leaving you vulnerable to disease and accelerated aging on the inside and outside.

Few people can weather and wear stress well. While you may not so easily see clogged arteries, high blood pressure, and abdominal fat, for example, in someone, you can usually see the signs of stress in her appearance, which is partly why I wholeheartedly believe that the elements of my program will help you to achieve better health overall, not just on the outside. For now, let's keep the focus on the skin. It will be the starting point from which all paths to wellness commence. And, as you're about to learn, the skin is in many ways its own command center that can talk to not only the brain but to other organs as well. So imagine the power you can wield on your beauty if *you* can command your skin and brain.

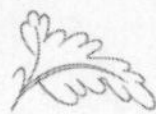

The Moms Who Changed Everything By the late '90s, many researchers were convinced that stress leads to chronic problems like heart disease, impaired immunity, memory loss, and premature aging, but there was no absolute proof. Then, in November 2004, a study of moms changed everything.

A team of scientists, led by researchers from the University of California, San Francisco, tracked fifty-eight mothers, aged twenty to fifty. Almost forty of them were caregivers—mothers with a chronically ill child. The rest (the controls) had healthy children. Predictably, the caregivers reported more stress than the controls, and the longer they had been caring for a sick child, the greater their stress.

What made this study a landmark was that scientists actually pinpointed the damage stress does to DNA, the genetic material in every one of our cells. The tips of DNA strands are protected by little shields called *telomeres* (like plastic tips at the end of shoelaces). The more stress a mom had, the shorter her telomeres were.

Telomeres, the UCSF group discovered, turn out to be a kind of clock for gauging how old a cell is. Each time a cell divides, the telomere tips shrink a bit. A repair enzyme quickly fixes them, but only so many repairs can be done. And the more stress a person is under, the less well the repairs work. When the DNA is damaged beyond repair, the cell can no longer divide. End of story.

The scientists did some fancy calculations and finally wound up with a way to measure the aging effects of stress. The telomeres of women with the greatest stress were 10 years older than those of the women with the least stress.

The research is ongoing, and here's the upside: The UCSF team is now trying to figure out if it's possible to counter the effects of stress on telomeres with meditation, therapy, yoga, or some other technique.

Q: What do you do when you're stressed?

A: Listening to music often helps me. It's great that music is so portable today—you can briefly tune out and go into a feel-good song. It's a four-minute fix! A little Patti Griffin works for me. Or James Blunt or a Crosby, Stills, and Nash flashback. Or listening to something I loved from high school or college.

I'm also a huge fan of the great outdoors. A dip in nature can make my whole body relax. As you know, I call it getting my vitamin G. When I'm tense, if I can go outside for even five minutes, it helps. I also practice what I preach about deep breathing: When I need to quickly chill out, I'll slowly breathe in through my nose and out through my mouth for a minute or two. I'll also mentally put myself in the last place I had a great vacation or was able to really relax. I tap into all my senses and focus on what the place looked like, smelled like, sounded like, and felt like. It helps me reset my emotions.

To understand how the mind-beauty connection works and why your skin needs certain ingredients to look its best, it helps to get a basic idea of how skin operates on the inside. Next up is a crash course.

6

skinology

Anatomy of Skin and the Seven Ways Stress Can Mess with Your Looks

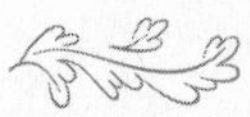

Because so many well-formulated beauty lines exist out there today that work well for the vast majority of people, I'm a lot less likely to see skin problems caused by products than skin problems triggered by stress. When I see a full-scale acne breakout on a patient who has rarely had a single pimple in the past, I first explain that acne is the *symptom,* not the problem (making for a long appointment with me). Over-the-brink stress can also show up as sudden hair loss in women, or I'll hear a patient lament, "I did not have this wrinkle last week" or "I look ten years older than I did three months ago." With a little sage (doable!) advice and direction from me, they make the connection and realize that the stress, sleeplessness, and anxiety are ruining their looks, accelerating their aging like gasoline on a fire, and maybe setting them up for depression, too.

It's amazing to think that what goes on up in the brain can have such an impact on our appearance, but guess what: What goes on in our skin can also have a huge impact. Your brain and skin are like twins in so many ways, and the things science is currently uncovering about their special relationship are astounding. Let's take a tour.

your skin: behind the scenes

You think *you've* got a lot to juggle? Skin is the ultimate multitasker, by design. Its major function? Playing gatekeeper to the outside world, shutting out invading viruses, bacteria, and toxins. But it also keeps tabs on the scene inside your body, fighting off infections, warming you up, cooling you down, and keeping you moist (90 percent of you and 70 percent of your skin is water). Skin also sometimes acts like a sponge, absorbing the sun's UVB rays, which help the body manufacture vitamin D for jobs like bone building and maintaining the nervous system.

Skin Fact

Our skin is our largest organ, taking up about 16 percent of our total body weight. It contains hair, oil and sweat glands, nerves, and blood vessels.

Your skin is also

- a communications specialist, silently telegraphing health or illness, pleasure or pain, embarrassment or enthusiasm
- a total-body outfit . . . the means by which you touch and feel everything (and are touched, as in, *mmm*, massage)
- a shock absorber, insulator, and wound healer
- one of the few organs that regenerates itself: Skin sheds dead cells and grows new ones continually, totally renewing itself every four to five weeks.

Like a beautiful cross-section of a multitiered layered cake, the skin is an amazing concoction of layers that is both fragile and strong. Some layers are moist and delicate, others are rich and sturdy; each supports the ones above it. However, if one layer is off, it can undermine the whole effect, making the surface sag or the texture dry or the colors all wrong. Disruptions can come from the outside world, too: Allergy-provoking toxins and acne-flaring hormones are the skin's equivalent of too much heat, overbeating, or bad ingredients.

Internal versus External Skin Aging

The skin, like all other organs, undergoes chronological aging and environmental aging. Stress aging can have an impact on both: It can accelerate internal aging as well as exacerbate external aging. Chronological aging, otherwise called *intrinsic* or *endogenous* aging, depends on the passage of time and is influenced by your genetics, hormonal changes, and metabolic processes. Habits like smoking cigarettes, drinking too much alcohol, and of course, having too much stress, can also factor into your chronological aging. This kind of aging can be seen on body areas not exposed to UV sunlight, and can reflect the aging process taking place in internal organs. Aged skin in nonexposed areas shows typical characteristics including fine wrinkles, dryness, sallowness, and loss of elasticity.

Environmental skin aging, on the other hand, is exactly that, aging accelerated by the elements you encounter from the outside world. This can entail UV radiation from the sun, but also air pollution, invasions of pathogens like bacteria and viruses, chemicals, and mechanical stress (e.g., constant tugging and pulling, as in the small crease you've got to the right of your mouth because you favor that side when you smile). Of all these external sources of age accelerators, UV radiation is the most influential one. Also called *photoaging,* it can damage the skin to such an extent that the skin prematurely ages. For this reason, you'll find that many of my strategies and skin recipes on the program (and that I hope you will adopt forever) help to treat UV damage and prevent further damage.

Thin Skin Fact

During internal aging, the skin gradually loses its structural and functional characteristics. Anatomically, the epidermis undergoes thinning by 10 to 50 percent between the age of thirty and eighty years, although the number of the cell layers remains the same.

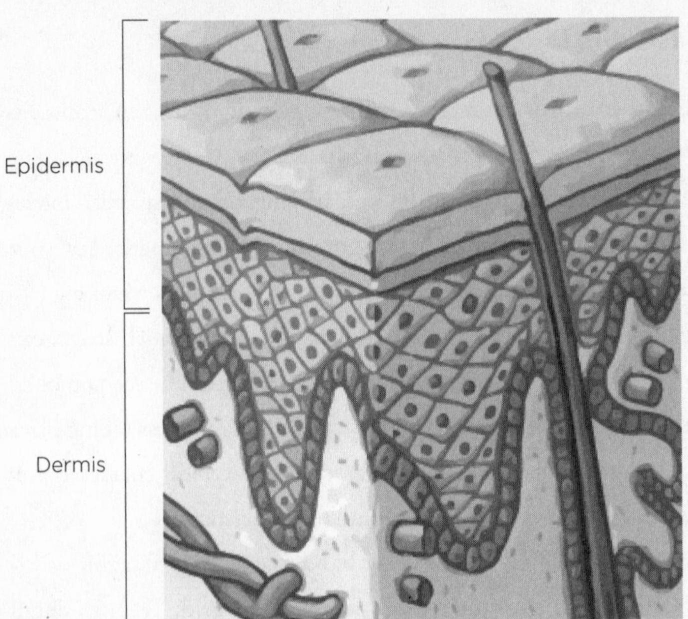

A section of the skin's upper layers.

skinography: a quick tour

While it helps to think of skin as a cake with multiple layers from a structural standpoint, from a *mechanical* perspective, the skin acts more like a large, multilevel manufacturing plant. It requires a certain supply of materials, including fuel, to keep the assembly lines operating and the overall system working efficiently. Most people don't realize all that can be found in skin. Skin isn't just skin, as in a collection of one type of cell. Much to the contrary, skin holds an array of compounds so it can do its job. These include proteins, amino acids, water, vitamins, trace minerals, antioxidants, fats, and sugar. In addition to protecting you against foreign invaders from the outside world, it also must protect itself by keeping its structures intact, hydrated, and healthy. It's a hungry and thirsty machine that needs more and more input and maintenance as you age because, like any machine, it becomes more inefficient and less reliable with time and constant use.

The First Layer

Let's start at the very bottom with the foundation: a layer of *subcutaneous fat*, which provides energy storage and protective padding, cushioning flesh and bones when you slip on ice, for instance. It also insulates your body from heat and cold, and it's the starting point for these other vital skin components.

- Sweat glands—they filter out toxins, water, and excess salt and are an essential part of your air-conditioning system. As sweat evaporates, it cools your jets. These glands start here but like any good AC system, they spiral upward.
- Lymphatics and blood vessels—they permeate the foundation layer, sending and receiving messages (you know: "ahhh, that feels nice," "wow, that's cold," "ouch!"), delivering nourishment, and providing transport and cleanup crews for cuts and infections. As with the sweat glands, they extend upward into the next layer, like zillions of tiny staircases.

What happens naturally as you age. Your skin's fat layer shrinks. Without that extra insulation, you feel the heat and cold more keenly, and your cheeks look more hollowed. (So why doesn't fat disappear from other parts of your anatomy too, like, say, your belly and hips? Sorry, but that's a different kind of fat.)

The Midlayers

This is the *dermis*, the largest layer of skin (accounting for about 90 percent of skin). It provides the struts and beams that add structure, strength, and elasticity, thanks to sturdy, protein-based connective tissue made of thin, white collagen fibers and wavy, rubbery, branching elastin fibers. Elastin holds the collagen together. This mesh of fibers forms the skin's infrastructure and gives it strength and resilience. Nearby, fibroblasts constantly churn out these two fibers. Unluckily, production slows down over time, and quality control gets sloppy, too. It's been theorized that these fibroblasts, as well as other cells, have a finite number of times they can divide. And when division comes to a halt, guess what: You age.

There are other things in these rich layers, including *sebaceous* or oil glands. These produce *sebum*, an oily, moisture-loving substance that helps keep skin soft. Hair follicles are located here as well; each one grows a single hair, varying in thickness from coarse eyebrows to the downy fuzz that senses you're about to be touched even before you actually are.

Right above these are water-loving ingredients called *glycosaminoglycans* (GAGs for short) that help moisturize skin and bolster collagen. Hyaluronic acid is a dominating GAG that surrounds the collagen-elastin network, binding it together and helping to keep the skin moist and plump. As you age, levels of hyaluronic acid decline, making the skin less pliable, drier, and gaunt. Additional blood and lymph vessels and nerve endings inhabit these two layers as well.

The dermis takes center stage in keeping your skin hydrated. The fact it's comprised of about 60 percent water and a gel-like mix of various molecules designed to nourish and hold moisture says a lot. Most of the signs of aging we all see in people are happening in this layer.

What happens naturally as you age. As Bette Davis said, growing old ain't for sissies. Fibroblasts decrease in number, and fewer fibroblasts mean less collagen and elastin, and that means the internal scaffolding begins to get shaky and skin loses its bounce-back-ability. Add in the millions of times you've smiled, frowned, winked, and yawned—no one keeps a totally straight face—and you've etched in a grid of furrows and wrinkles. Fat shrinkage beneath the surface contributes to deeper folds. Skin tends to become drier over time, too, especially after menopause, partly because oil and sweat production slow and partly due to hormonal changes—an effect stress can mimic, by the way, but we'll get to that later.

In addition, the skin's water-holding GAGs decrease with age so there is a lot less moisture to go around. It's a double whammy: The tough, fibrous collagen-elastic matrix weakens and the nearby hydrating molecules decrease in volume. Thus, there's less water around to keep the collagen and elastic flexible and moist. The drought further affects new cells developing, as well as the dead cells on the skin's surface.

Finally, skin becomes paler, because its supply of blood vessels diminishes. Blood vessels are necessary for transporting nutrients and moisture, and removing cellular waste. When an area of the skin loses its access to critical ingredients it needs to stay renewed, hydrated, and nourished; it begins to show the signs of aging. Smoking and sun damage will worsen this scenario. Smoking will suffocate your skin, limiting its access to oxygen. UV rays from the sun will cause blood vessel walls to thicken, and as the blood vessels dilate, they become visible as tiny red threads just below the surface. They may also twist and break.

The Upper Layers

Now we've reached the skin areas that are closest to the light above—the layers of the *epidermis*. The epidermis has a love-hate relationship with the outside world: It pulls in water, heat, and light, and pushes away bacteria, dirt, germs, and toxins.

- *Keratinocytes* are the primary players here. These plump cells form at the base of the epidermis and flatten out as they rise to the surface, die, and eventually flake off. Ironically, these dead cells, collectively known as the *stratum corneum*, make up what we call our skin—the birthday suit we touch, wash, dry, pamper, and protect (even if we sometimes pierce or tattoo it).

- Keratinocytes produce *keratin*, which is the same tough protein that's in hair and fingernails; on the skin's surface, it helps form a roadblock against would-be intruders.

- Tough-guy immune system forces called *Langerhans' cells* are located here, too; they detect foreign substances. More than that, recently these cells have gained greater recognition as extraordinary players in immunity. In late 2005, researchers at Yale School of Medicine demonstrated that Langerhans' cells in the skin, which had been thought to alert the immune system to invaders, instead dampen the skin's reaction to infection and inflammation. We now view these cells not just as sentinels or stimulators of immune reactions as previously thought, but more as environmental peacekeepers. The skin is constantly challenged by the environment, but most challenges are not dangerous and do not warrant an immune response. Your Langerhans try to keep the peace before warranting a full-fledged response.
- *Melanocytes* churn out *melanin*, which determines the color of your skin, that is, whether you're dark or pale. It's the pigment that protects skin from too much ultraviolet light by darkening it after repeated UV exposure, at least in some people. Some types of melanin (Irish-Americans know this all too well) are simply too light to provide any UV protection.

What happens naturally as you age. Your body makes less of all this good stuff, which translates into more challenges. Less melanin (melanocytes drop off by 10 to 20 percent every decade) means more susceptibility to UV rays, more brown spots (white spots too, in some people), more wrinkling, a paler overall appearance, and a higher risk of skin cancer. Hence every skin doc's mantra for her patients: sunscreen, shade, hats, and more sunscreen. Also, the top layer thins, becoming a less effective barrier to bad guys from the outside and moisture loss from the inside. And the number of immune defenders, those Langerhan's cells, drops off, which makes skin extra vulnerable to infection and cancer.

That ends the minitour of your skin and what happens to it naturally with age, what's known as *intrinsic aging. Extrinsic aging* is what doesn't happen to it naturally. Surely you know that certain habits can influence the speed of your natural aging. Most of these factors, fortunately, are things you can try to control—smoking, tanning, deciding whether to choose Mick Jagger or Denise Austin as a role model. Making healthy choices could win you the Hasn't Changed a Bit! award at your twenty-fifth reunion. But as you've figured out by now, it's not all physical. In fact, age and beauty is very much a mental match between two brains—the one in your head and *the one in your skin.*

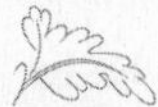

The Skin Stress Test One place where stress takes an invisible toll is on the skin's role as a barrier between you and the world. Researchers have a clever way of testing this. They injure skin slightly by repeatedly applying and pulling off a piece of cellophane tape from a small area. (Sounds painful, but isn't really.) They then watch how quickly it recovers by measuring the amount of moisture that seeps out of the irritated area. When a team of scientists did this test on healthy women, they found that two stresses—sleep deprivation and a mock job interview—significantly held up the skin's recovery. However, exercising on a treadmill didn't slow it a whit. If that's what happens in the lab, think of what happens in real life, when sleepless nights are often the norm and a job interview is the least of your pressures.

skin has a mind of its own

One of the most provocative and exciting discoveries in the last decade is that skin also has its own stress-response system. Just as our central body as a whole (in medical terms, we refer to this as *systemic*) has a brilliant system set up to handle stressful situations, our skin has its own local, fully functional equivalent. In other words, the skin has established its own independent, yet parallel version of the hypothalamic-pituitary-adrenal axis. It can produce forms of the same molecules famously manufactured and used by the central body during a stressful event, including ACTH and CRH, cortisol, beta-endorphin, as well as serotonin and melatonin—two hormones key to mood. It's amazing to think that skin is not only an unexpectedly prominent target organ for multiple signals, which have a profound impact on its health and risk for disease, but also an astonishing *factory* for the same signals. Our skin and nervous system share a language we are just beginning to understand. And, in fact, the field of medicine devoted to translating this complex language is one of the fastest-moving, most exciting, branches of skin research.

Skin's Twin

Your skin and entire nervous system, including your brain, share the same embryological origin in the ectoderm, a germ layer when you were just a bundle of initial cells. No wonder the two share similar hormones and neurotransmitters. They are practically twins.

Hardly any other organ is continuously exposed to such a wide range of stressors as the skin. Twenty-four hours a day, over our entire lifetime, the skin remains our interface with the world, so it's easy to see how it must be exquisitely well designed, innervated, and self-sufficient to a degree. It not only reacts to your real brain's red alerts but it actually orchestrates its own network of messages. When the skin is under attack—by the sun's UV rays, for instance—certain skin cells release CRH, the messenger that the brain puts in charge when stress shows up. Likewise, cortisol, which rushes out from the adrenal glands in a crisis, can also be produced in the skin by pigment cells and hair follicles.

How could the skin be so smart? For starters, skin has always shared a unique bond with the brain and central nervous system. Let's cast back to a time when you were nothing but a small bundle of cells (no, not a bundle of joy yet; I'm talking about when you were just an embryo of only a few weeks old). Back then, you consisted of two distinct layers: an outer *ectoderm* and an inner *endoderm*. The *ecto*dermal cells gave rise to your entire nervous system (which includes your brain, spinal cord, and peripheral nerves), portions of special sensory organs, outer skin and its glands, hair, nails, and linings of the mouth and anal canal. The *endo*dermal cells, on the other hand, became the outer linings of your digestive tract, respiratory tract, urinary bladder, and urethra. (Another layer, called the *mesoderm*, which grows soon *after* these two first layers, is what forms all types of interior tissues like muscle, bone, blood, lymph, and the lining of the body cavities.)

I've been deeply fascinated by this since high school biology. It's not very intuitive to think that your skin, which is thought of as being on the *outside*, shares its beginnings with the brain and nervous system, which are thought of as being on the *inside*. It's hard to picture your brain and nervous system as being on your outside, but remember that we're talking about the very early stage of life when you were an embryo and far from looking the way you do today. So, while the brain essentially started as an outer layer on you when you were just a ball of cells, it eventually folded inward, leaving your developing skin layer (in good hands on its own!) to fend for itself on the outside. That's quite a close relationship to have from the beginning. No wonder the skin and brain share such close personal ties, and can act like each other in a lot of ways.

Think about what it means from an evolutionary perspective, though, to have your skin and brain so intimately connected. If you were in danger, and your skin got wind of this first (let's say, when a sneaky saber-toothed tiger tried to take a bite out of your hand while you were looking the other way), wouldn't it be ideal for your skin to have the ability to respond on its own quickly rather than wait for your brain to send the signal? In other words, when you retract your hand and leap as far back as you can from the beast, you can thank your *skin* first, and your brain second.

Now, that may be oversimplifying what happens at the cellular level, but the point is our skin's ability to act in many ways like our brains isn't a fluke. It's rooted in our survival mechanisms, which have been encoded in us since the dawn of humans. The skin is our first line of defense against the potentially dangerous outer world where we are vulnerable to injury, illness, and disease. It makes total sense that skin can signal to, and inspire, the brain to take action. I've always wondered, for example, why it can seemingly take a few moments to feel pain when you stub your toe. The skin reacts fast, as you feel the pressure and watch the area swell with blood and bruising. But perhaps the physical sensation of pain is delayed because the brain needs that extra blip of time to get the message that your toe is injured. Something to think about—literally.

We are just beginning to decode this complex intersystem communication that intimately meshes the body's largest and most external organ with the endocrine, nervous, and immune systems. The fact that skin can produce some of the same substances once thought to be exclusive to the brain and nervous system, and the fact that skin, as a pivotal immune agent, can initiate immune responses on its very own (as opposed to waiting for the brain to take action) is nothing short of extraordinary. The skin has its own flight-or-flight response system independent of the brain. What this also means, however, is that skin can instigate responses that result in unwanted outcomes, such as acne, rashes, and troubling skin conditions. In addition, the messages that come firing out from the skin locally or through the central nervous system can have a direct effect on the production of beauty-promoting collagen and elastin. Certain stress responses will halt or slow down their growth. We'll be taking a look at how this happens shortly.

This gives whole new meaning to the notion that you look how you feel. Contrary to popular belief, skin is not passive and it's not just about the barrier function.

Calling All Skin Cells! The back-and-forth signaling system between your central body and skin, as well as *within* your skin alone, is like your body's own wireless network. The communications happen thanks to small chains of amino acids called peptides, which facilitate the talking that goes on between cells. Neuropeptides originate in the nervous system and brain (hence, the *neuro* part), including the peripheral nerve endings in skin. One neuropeptide that gets a lot of attention in research circles is called Substance P. It's a well-known chemical that promotes pain in the body, and can also increase sebum production (not a good thing if you're prone to acne). Substance P may further be a player in depression and anxiety, which are often affiliated with acne.

When the body senses stress, nerves, especially nerve endings in the skin, send out Substance P in response. When neuropeptide receptors in skin receive messages, they react by sharing the message out to other cells, which tells them how to function. This is how the feeling of embarrassment can move from your brain to your skin, causing it to blush. Similarly, when you are happy, your skin glows; you are white as a ghost when frightened. It's as if we were chameleons and can change pretty quickly; what we are thinking and how we are feeling has an outward appearance.

And by the same token, how the *skin* thinks and feels determines what goes on locally, too. Environmental stress factors such as pollutants, heat, allergens, high or low humidity, and mechanical stretching can usher Substance P as well as other peptides locally to take action. When external trouble starts, it has to throw up defenses and put its repair crews on alert *fast*. What's more, the production of collagen and elastin in skin reflects the activity of these peptides. Certain messages will either halt or encourage collagen and elastin growth, thus leading to either youthful-looking skin or a prunish appearance. These messages will also affect other systems that factor into our appearance, such as how much blood flows to the skin, fostering a healthy glow or a pallid look.

Skin Is Big and Nervous

The skin boasts a lot of number ones: It's the largest organ in terms of size, and has the biggest nerve supply of any organ in the body. (Trivia: Your fingertips win for being the most nervous region of your skin. Those little digits receive approximately 300 impulses [technically, mechanoreceptive nerve fibers] per square centimeter!) No wonder we call ourselves "touchy" and "feely."

seven sneaky ways stress can mess with your looks

Given what you've learned thus far, it's not hard to draw the connections and understand how chronic stress can affect how you look. Let's explore seven big conclusions.

Stress Can Cause Wrinkles

Recall that cortisol degrades collagen. When you consider what exactly a wrinkle is—a weakening and lessening of collagen and elastin fibers in the skin's dermis—it's easy to understand how stress, then, can directly cause wrinkles. When you live in a chronic state of stress, routinely bathing your body in cortisol, it becomes harder and harder for the skin to repair itself naturally, continue to form healthy collagen and elastin, and deal with damaged areas. At the same time, your body is responding to the stress through inflammatory pathways, which can exacerbate skin issues.

But here's the good news: If you can decrease your levels of cortisol and increase your levels of beta-endorphins, which act as anti-inflammatories in the body as well as in skin, you can reverse this damage. And that's exactly what you are doing on this program. It's a win-win when you can control your cortisol levels and maximize your beta-endorphins. How do you increase your beta-endorphins? Restful sleep and frequent sex and exercise are three great ways, which is why they are highlighted during the nine days.

It's important to remember, too, that aging is simply a process by which your capacity to repair tissues and manufacture fresh new cells declines. What we want to do is tip the scales in favor of slowing down that natural decline, as well as boost the speed of cellular repair. Beta-endorphins retard that decline, and controlling cortisol levels keeps the repair shop clear of this villain that will do more damage.

I had a woman come to me in her fifties who proclaimed how much better and younger she felt now than ten years previously, when her life was out of balance. She had gone from being a diehard trial lawyer—working crazy hours, forgoing sleep, and avoiding exercise—to becoming a new mother. Having the baby instantly changed her life (not to mention priorities), because with the baby came the need to take better care of herself first, if she was to be a good mom and still handle the rigors of her daily life. She explained that no sooner did she begin to make a few lifestyle changes than she began to see a noticeable difference in her looks and energy level. When she showed me a photo of her old self from ten years earlier, it was stunning to see the transformation. She had come to me for a full body check and to make sure she had a plan for staying as young as possible, especially since she was taking on motherhood at a time when her friends were becoming grandparents. I told her she was well on her way to preserving her good looks and vitality just by having a more balanced life now.

Stress Can Bring on Nasty Adult Acne

Acne isn't just for hormonally crazed teenagers anymore. Many adults can't seem to outgrow it because of stress hormones. Yet most people don't make the connection. They come into my office asking whether it's their chocolate habit (no), or if their skin has somehow gotten oilier (not likely), or whether their soap, makeup, or moisturizer could be to blame (possibly, but not probably).

If there's simply too much going on in their lives, odds are it's stress acne and CRH is the culprit. Acne *is* an inflammatory condition and CRH has already been linked to other inflammatory disorders. Also, the skin's own production of CRH may fuel inflammation that leads to acne. What can make things worse is that tense people often can't leave pimples alone. Squeezing, poking, and picking at them becomes an almost obsessive way to release tension, but it also makes breakouts worse, exacerbating the inflammatory response, and you're left feeling a tad more stressed. It's one of those vicious cycles. When you add a wrinkle or two to that, you've got a cocktail of frustration. I see more patients who complain of both pimples and wrinkles than people who complain of one of those two things alone. And luckily there is something you can do about it. You're not stuck living with skin not knowing whether you're sixteen or forty-six.

I've devoted an entire section to acne in chapter 8 so hang tight.

Stress Can Make Your Skin Irritated and Allergic

Your skin has mast cells, which release *histamines* in response to biochemicals like stress hormones. Histamines are key players in allergies and inflammation; they can trigger ailments like hay fever and asthma, and in the skin they can wreak havoc on skin disorders and disease. These mast cells are located right near blood vessels and nerve endings, and they can be activated by a plethora of biochemicals, chiefly those classic stress hormones ACTH and CRH. Scientists now believe that mast cells are among the richest source of CRH outside the brain. What's more, mast cells have the capacity to generate CRH *on their own*, so imagine the damage they can do when they run amok. Once triggered through the biochemical pathways—by anger, depression, pain, pollutants, UV light, free radicals, heat, cold, or any mind/body stressors—mast cells can stir up a soup of chemical pests. These, in turn, can set off a range of skin conditions or simply aggravate existing ones, from dermatitis and hives to psoriasis and even hair loss. And because your skin talks to your brain and vice versa, something like a nasty itch can ratchet up your entire body's stress levels and keep you in a cycle of inflammation and irritation.

There's some early evidence that when skin gets inflamed by stress, including simple sun exposure, it forms more nerve fibers, which makes it even more sensitive and may contribute to photoaging. Put simply, the more the skin is exposed to certain stress hormones, the more receptors your skin will have to perpetuate a reaction. Stress, even if it's just psychological, can trigger a physical change in neuronal connections.

Stress Can Make Your Hair Fall Out and Your Nails Brittle

When I was in college, a friend of mine experienced sudden hair loss about three months into her freshman year. Her hair was on her clothes, bedding, and personal items. It wasn't coming out in clumps, and she wasn't balding in any specific area, but her head was definitely shedding the hair at an alarming rate. She had arrived with a thick head of hair, but it became noticeably thinner by the time we all went home for Thanksgiving weekend. That's when she scheduled a visit with her doctor, hoping to find out she had a thyroid problem or some disorder that would have a quick fix.

Her physician found nothing wrong with her and recommended she see a dermatologist, which she did right away. That's when she got the bad news: Most of the hairs on her head were in the resting, or telogen, phase of the hair cycle. At any given time, a random number of hairs will be in various stages of growth and shedding. Her doctor had plucked a few strands to examine the ends that came from the follicle. He noted that they had prematurely stopped growing and had entered into an inactive phase called the telogen phase. The culprit? While genetics could share some of the blame, especially given the fact she was eighteen years old—a time when the genes for hair loss could be turning on—the doctor pointed to stress as being the most likely cause. This was not good news for my friend, who was stressing out over her hair loss. Hearing that hair loss was a normal response to stress wasn't what she was hoping for. How does one stop stressing over a side effect of stress? This is when you need some serious mind-over-matter techniques.

Stress can cause sudden hair loss by literally flipping the switch on the hair follicle's growth stage from an active to a resting phase. Once the follicle enters this resting phase prematurely, it stays there for about three months, after which time a large amount of hair will be shed. Usually by then the person has recovered from the stressful event so she will regain a new head of hair. Women who go through pregnancy and experience sudden hair loss about three months after childbirth can blame their hormones for that loss. Between

20 and 45 percent of mothers lose hair after giving birth as their estrogen and progesterone levels drop, and hair follicles are thrust into the inactive phase. Luckily, most mothers will regain their head of hair nine to twelve months after the child's birth (assuming they get a good handle on their stress levels caused by a baby).

More recently, when a patient came to me complaining of sudden hair loss, I immediately asked her what happened in her life over the previous six months. Turns out she had a medical scare when doctors found a spot on her lung and thought it was cancer. She had prepared for the worst and went through all the emotions of possibly having to deal with lung cancer. It wasn't cancer in the end, so she thought she had gotten over it quickly. When I explained that this experience likely spun her hair follicles into a resting phase prematurely, and that her hair would come back with time, she was relieved. It helped her tremendously to understand that the lag time between the crisis in life and the hair loss can be confusing. When you experience an overall shedding of hair (your hairbrush fills up and the drain gets clogged in the shower every day), you must cast back a few months to find the trigger. And rest assured that you can recover your hair when it grows back. Just knowing that can take the stress out!

Now if gray hair is a problem, that's another issue largely determined by genetics. Whether or not extreme stress, especially the psychoemotional kind, can turn hair prematurely gray is a contested area of study. Stress has been shown to affect melanocytes in hair follicles, which are responsible for giving your hair color. No one goes gray overnight, though, contrary to old wives' tales. Researchers are now finding that stress may have detrimental effects on melanocyte *stem* cells, suggesting this could result in permanent damage that contributes to stress-induced graying. Researchers are also finding that hair follicle stem cells that are vital for maintenance and the cyclic renewal of hair growth may also fall prey to irreversible damage and bring on more serious types of hair loss such as alopecia areata. People who have this condition experience hair loss in clumps and have round hairless patches on the scalp. The immune system is also involved, as stress activates T-cells, which are part of your immune system and supposed to attack pathogens like viruses and bacteria. When activated, T-cells surround the follicles, they do so like a swarm of bees—effectively killing them. So it's as if stress becomes a pathogen, and your immune system goes on the attack, even though it's attacking *you*. We call this an autoimmune disease, and volumes of books could be written about the link between stress (even stress as simple as an emotional letdown) and autoimmune disorders. I think viewing stress as a pathogen in itself is a realistic way to look at it.

Q: Does excess and embarrassing hair on my face mean something is wrong with me?

A: Very unlikely. If you feel like you're growing a light beard and face new hairs every morning, especially on your chin, see your doctor. This could potentially be a problem involving your adrenal glands; or it could be polycystic ovarian syndrome, a disorder whereby high levels of male hormones get pumped out. But, more than likely, you can thank your genes for excessive hair and there is absolutely nothing wrong with you! What I think is wrong, however, is the means by which too many women try to remove the hair—shaving. Never shave your face; it's demoralizing for a woman and will dampen your feminine spirit. If you've had it with waxing and plucking, then consider laser hair removal. Prescription creams that retard hair growth are also available, but laser hair removal will nip your hairs in the bud forever. You may have to schedule a monthly electrolysis session for up to a year, but then you'll never have to fight those unsightly follicles again.

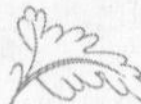

Hair Razing Fact Sudden stress-related hair loss characterized by a general thinning throughout the entire scalp is called *telogen effluvium*. Stress can literally shock hair follicles into an inactive state, after which they will likely fall out. This is seen more in women because pregnancy is one such event that can trigger this kind of hair loss. It's not so much that pregnancy itself is überstressful on the body (although the *physical* stress on the stretched-out skin is what causes those lovely stretch marks!), but the hormonal changes can affect a head of hair. Pregnant women may notice thicker and healthier hair during their pregnancy, attributed to the increased levels of hormones estrogen and progesterone. But after the baby is born, those hormone levels drop rapidly, triggering a shift from active to resting phases in the follicles. Then out comes the hair about three months later. Coupled with the drop in hormone levels at the birth of a child is, of course, the general stress that a new mother experiences, all of which bodes poorly on those precious hair follicles.

Nails are not resistant to stress of the physical kind. Brittle, peeling nails also are a common side effect of traumatic stress, chiefly the kind caused by repeated wetting and drying, and chronic exposure to detergents, water, toluene and formaldehyde in polish, and harsh solvents (like those found in nail polish remover). Other factors could also be at play, including genes, poor diet, and underlying medical conditions. Let's not forget the fact that many try to cope with psychological stress by self-inflicting hair and nail problems (skin, too) that go beyond what I would normally expect from stress alone. For example, how many of us find ourselves rigorously biting or picking at our nails when we are nervous, anxious, or stressed out maximally? How many of us pick at our skin or consistently touch and play with acne and flareups? Do you pull on your hair to the point you feel a few strands fall out? It's important to note these habits and take steps to avoid engaging in these beauty-busting behaviors. Like the eyes, nails can say a lot about your health and how well you take care of yourself.

Filing Down a Nail Myth Contrary to popular belief, our nails do not contain much calcium, so supplementation, while good for our bones, may not help our nails. In fact, vitamin and mineral deficiencies are rare causes of nail problems. More often than not, brittle nails are caused by excessive exposure to harsh soaps, irritants, polish remover, and the wetting and drying of nails (all typical of a busy, kitchen-maven mom). Brittle nails can also be seen with medical conditions like psoriasis, fungal infections, and thyroid problems. Age also factors in, and the older you are the more likely your nails will become brittle.

That said, one little nutrient that may help give your nails a boost is *biotin*. Found abundantly in foods like cauliflower, peanuts, and lentils, biotin is absorbed into the core of the nail, where it may encourage a better, thicker nail to grow and help prevent splitting and cracking. In one study, people who consumed 2.5 milligrams of biotin daily had marked increases in nail thickness after six months. To get this much biotin, ask your doctor about taking it in supplement form.

Hangnail Hangup

What causes a hangnail? The culprit is a cuticle that gets too dry and splits off. When a hangnail sprouts, carefully trim it so you're not tempted to peel it. You can also help it out by applying a topical antibiotic like Neosporin; this will kill the bacteria and hydrate the skin. Preventing hangnails is all about keeping your cuticles moisturized. You can use any cream to do this, and push back your cuticles once a week.

Stress Can Affect Your Hormones, Which in Turn Affect Your Mood, and Vice Versa

The biochemistry of mood and how it affects our physiology is a fascinating topic, and one we've already covered with talk about cortisol, in particular. There is a lot of interaction between hormone physiology and mood that works both ways. Our mood can impact our physiology, and our physiology can influence the balance of our hormones. Additionally, our body can *interpret* our mood—anger, sadness, exhaustion, and so on—as, you guessed it, stress.

Take, for example, tiredness. It's late at night and you haven't been getting much sleep lately. You're irritable and feel like you've just tied the end of your rope and are now hanging on. Not only has your level of stress caused a surge in cortisol, which can trip your appetite, but chances are your body's balance of appetite hormones—namely *leptin* and *ghrelin*—will also be out of whack, so you'll crave sugary, high-calorie foods. This is when you rummage through your refrigerator for last night's chocolate cake, topping it off with mac-and-cheese leftovers from your kids' dinner. Then the guilt sets in, and you hate yourself for gorging so late at night on fattening food. When you notice that you're up a tick or two on the scale the next day, *that* stresses you out some more. The cycle continues the next night when you stare at the ceiling stressing about all sorts of things, from your weight gain to your unfinished chores and bad mood that resulted in a fight with your husband after dinner.

Lost in Translation

You may be extremely uptight and worried about making a presentation at work or confronting your spouse about a sensitive issue, and while you may call yourself *anxious*, your body will say *stressed*. You cannot divorce mood and emotions from hormones and stress, so let's get a handle on them!

Don't blame yourself. Food and mood go hand in hand, and sometimes we have our own biochemistry to thank for how we behave. Two other hormones I want to mention before moving on, especially as they relate to mood, are serotonin and melatonin. Technically, these are not stress hormones, but they do get involved in the stress cycle by virtue of the fact they affect how we feel. *Serotonin* is our pleasure hormone, and its strong connection to mood and emotion is why drugs to treat depression help elevate the levels of serotonin in the brain. Levels can be affected by many factors, including stress hormones, chemicals in the foods we eat, sleep deprivation, and the amount of sunlight we get in a day. Low serotonin and melatonin levels in the brain are thought to be contributing factors to depression. *Mel-*

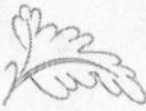

The Bigger Picture The hypothalamus is often referred to as the *seat of the emotions*. It takes center stage in emotional processing; the moment we even think about something stressful or encounter a stressful experience, the hypothalamus secretes CRH, which eventually leads to cortisol rushing out of the adrenal glands. Here's one way to see the big picture on how influential hormones can be once stress triggers the release of this master of ceremonies: cortisol leads to collagen and muscle breakdown, fat retention, hunger leads to overeating, sleep loss leads to exhaustion, moodiness, lack of control at the dinner table leads to more sleep loss, more stress, more weight gain, more collagen breakdown leads to wrinkles, baggy eyes, breakouts, poor diet choices leads to more frustration when we realize that now were overtired, overweight, moody, and looking haggard.

---

atonin is also a brain chemical related to mood but this one has closer ties to sleep; it serves as the body's main regulator of sleep-wake cycles. It may also be linked to several other aspects of physiology and consciousness.

The point of all this is to show you just how intertwined our moods and physiology can be. Every second of the day, your body's endocrine system choreographs a complex dance between glands and target organs to effect certain changes. As these changes occur, your physiology shifts, which can affect how you actually feel. Volumes of books could be written on hormonal physiology alone, even as it relates to stress. My goal here is to simply show you a few examples of how hormones shape what we do and how we feel. If stress can sit at the top of a cascade of events that lead to undesirable hormonal changes in the body (like those that trigger insomnia, insatiable hunger and weight gain, and collagen breakdown), then what we want to do is find ways to gain the upper hand on our stress level and ensure we foster an environment in our body that keeps all those hormones in check—in balance. And again, that is what the program helps you to achieve.

Stress Can Make Your Eyes Look Old

When someone says you look tired, you might feel the urge to slap him or her across the face. Seriously, the person is probably referring to your eyes, and not getting enough sleep is mostly to blame. Stress ages eyes by robbing us of deep, slow-wave sleep, the superrestorative kind that's essential to the youth and health of our whole body. Recall that it's during deep sleep that growth hormone gets released in the body to go to work on repairing and replenishing your cells. Blame CRH, too, which (among other things) acts like a stimulant, keeping you up at night. In short, getting too little shuteye sets off a series of skin problems—inflammation, leaky capillaries, and poor waste removal. Fluids that should be carted away while you sleep never get picked up, sort of like what happens when the trash collectors don't show up and the garbage gets overloaded. In your face, the excess liquid has to go somewhere, so it pools in the delicate tissue under the eyes. The result? Dark, puffy, under-eye circles.

Stress May Drive Your Skin into a Mini-menopause

The jury is still out on exactly how or if this is possible, but it's worth mentioning even if you're years away from the real thing happening. It appears that the constant flow of cortisol that goes along with chronic stress causes a dip in estrogen, one that mimics, on a smaller scale, the dip that occurs during menopause. And if you're already in menopause, the dip in estrogen can actually *increase* cortisol! That's something to think about considering that we now spend a third of our lives in menopause.

With less estrogen around, the three main ingredients that keep skin moist—basically, sweat glands, oil producers, and the superlubricator hyaluronic acid—slow their flow. Less estrogen means less collagen and less moisture. So, while estrogen levels may not drop enough to shut down your period, stress may make them dip enough to make your skin look dull and dry.

Although it's not exactly clear why estrogen holds such sway over our skin, we know that women who take hormone replacement therapy can reverse these changes, helping skin regain its youthful strength: It becomes less than paper thin, blood flow to the skin improves, and collagen production rebounds. In one study collagen production was almost 50 percent higher in women taking hormones. The influence of estrogen on several body systems is well documented, but we're just beginning to understand this hormone's influence on skin and will likely see more studies done in the future.

Less Stress, Safer Sex

Low estrogen can put a damper on your sex life. And this isn't just about stressed-out women in menopause. Stressed-out women on birth control pills can also experience low estrogen levels, which can cause a thinning of the vulva—that area that includes the inner and outer lips, the clitoris, and the opening of the vagina, and its glands. If it gets too thin you could experience tearing during sex. Ouch! Yet one more reason to wipe out as much stress as you can.

While no one is recommending that most women take estrogen these days (or not yet, though this case isn't totally closed), that's not the point here. The point is anything that puts a significant damper on the flow of estrogen in your body will ultimately age your skin. Stress does that, which is a critical reason to learn how to tame it.

what can you do about all this?

First, don't feel overwhelmed. I've given you a lot of information in this chapter and some of it may have left you feeling like you can't get control of your body because so much of what goes on happens naturally. True, the human body seemingly has a mind of its own and, when you're faced with stress, it's impractical (and unrealistic) to think you can just say "Stop the cortisol!" and your adrenal glands will listen. However, I want you to see the bigger picture here. I've outlined a few sequences of events that happen when we respond poorly to stress and let it get to us. Suddenly, our battle with stress ends up being a battle for a restful night's sleep, a battle to lose and maintain weight, a battle to feel energetic, a battle to exercise, a battle to look vibrant, a battle to take proper care of ourselves, a battle to maintain our health. And a battle to be happy. Some of you may already be in this vicious cycle and it's time to break it.

My hope is that once you begin to establish better coping skills for handling stress, and begin to employ the techniques I've outlined to nourish and treat your body optimally both inside and out, you will discover a path to wellness and beauty. You will achieve sound sleep. A fresh, glowing appearance. Energy. Motivation to stay active. And peace of mind. The benefits that await you are infinite.

I'm here to tell you that you *can* shift the balance of power into your hands and support a healthy balance in your body simply by changing the way you strategize through life. This entails establishing a few new habits and kicking out some old ones, which is exactly what the program outlined in chapter 4 helps you to do. I know you can do this. You must, because the time has come to put mind over matter, literally. It will affect everything about you, from your neurology to your immunology. Scientists currently are studying everything from the physiology of meditating monks to the DNA of caretaking moms. You know that those bags under your eyes disappear when you've hopped off the hamster wheel and slept well for a week.

Why Women Live Longer Things aren't all bad! As stressed as we are, women still have the advantage over men when it comes to coping. New evidence? In most parts of the world women now live about *ten years* longer than men. New cause? Differences in how we respond to a brain chemical called *oxytocin,* suggests the latest stress research. Sometimes referred to as the *bonding hormone* or *love hormone,* oxytocin makes people (animals, too) care for each other. Sex (and masturbation) will trigger its release, but it also has ties to stressful situations. When the going gets rough, it helps people feel more connected and less frightened.

Here is where the sexes are not created equal. While both men and women release oxytocin in some stressful situations, in men, testosterone appears to block oxytocin, so they stay in edgy fight-or-flight mode. In women, however, estrogen enhances nurturing oxytocin, so under stress we may shift from fight or flight to a calmer state called *tend and befriend.* Oxytocin also tempers surges in blood pressure, heart rate, and cortisol levels.

The tend-and-befriend theory makes evolutionary sense. Eons ago, while men sprang into action to fight off a saber-toothed something, the women closed in to nurture and protect the babies, assuring survival. So, maybe it's no surprise that today when we are stressed to the max, rather than fighting or fleeing, we often turn to each other, seeking comfort and consolation. Survival just might depend on it.

7

the beauty buffet and bar

Optimum Diet Choices for Beautiful Skin

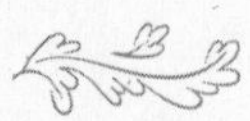

If I told you to go ahead and eat anything you want and you'll look beautiful no matter what, you would rejoice. Well, guess what: Having beautiful skin doesn't mean you have to do anything drastic to the way you eat. You can pretty much eat the way you always have. I'm only going to recommend that you make a few small shifts in your dietary habits and restrain from certain foods as much as possible.

I want you to gain an understanding of how food factors into this mind-beauty connection, and at least begin to take small steps that will help you achieve a healthier body overall, regardless of how much your diet factors into your physical looks. In this chapter, I'm going to share insights on the relationship between diet and beauty. And pardon the cliché, but you are what you eat. What you choose to consume says a lot about how you look and feel.

Fueling your body's engine with premium fuel helps fend off signs of aging in general, including wrinkles and dryness; eating well can even protect skin from sun damage. And let's be honest: Stress so often does a number on our eating habits. As I've said, and I trust you know from personal experience, when we are wired, fried, and moody, we are apt to reach for quick-fix foods (there's a real reason for this, so let go of the guilt). Over time, all those mocha lattes and Mars bars will expand our weight and waistline, boost our risk of heart disease, diabetes, stroke, and cancer, and add to our skin woes. That's a scenario for escalating stress, and *more* skin woes, if ever there were one!

One thing I want to get straight, though, is that I'm not here to act like an overbearing mother, forcing you to eat your vegetables, clean your plate, evict dessert from your life forever, and enter a zone of deprivation. How stressful would *that* be? The very nature of a diet equals stress to the body! And there are lots of gray areas in the food-face connection. Does chocolate really cause acne? Will stocking up on boatloads of salmon really ward off inflammation? Is there such a thing as a diet that guarantees clear skin? Those are among the questions I'm going to address.

First of all, if you haven't figured it out by now, we are complex beings. There is no magic pill, potion, or formula for beauty. Too many things coalesce in our bodies to produce either the results we want or don't want. You've already gotten a good dose of information about hormones, exercise, sleep, relaxation, deep breathing, and so on. Diet is yet another one to add to the mix. There is, however, plenty of scientific proof about eating certain foods to support your skin and health, while avoiding others that can sabotage your beauty goals. Don't panic: The point is not for you to do anything too unrealistic, such as suddenly savor wheatgrass juice or spoon flaxseed oil into your mouth every morning. You'll have *some* leeway.

Remember, this isn't about going on a specific diet. It's ultimately up to you to make modifications in how you eat so you can move over to a lifetime of healthy eating—and limitless beauty. As with any healthy eating guidelines, the goal here is to supply your cells and systems with the raw materials they need to function efficiently and optimally, inside and out. You don't want to give your body *any* excuse to age prematurely, so you need to be sure that at any given time it has all the resources it requires to stay alive, hydrated, and nourished to the max.

the skin-ny on the diet-beauty dilemma

A lot has been written lately about the diet-skin connection. There is definitely something to be said for how diet choices influence our blood chemistry, mood, and capacity to fight oxidative stress, free-radical production, and inflammation.

A book exploring the diet-skin connection, which is a giant field of study still in its infancy, is a book in itself. Much debate about this hot topic is currently under way, with doctors and researchers on both sides of the table trying to understand and decipher just how diet does, or does not, factor into the beauty equation. Because diet is something we can (or at least try to) control in our lives, it gives us great hope to think we can control our health and beauty through diet alone. But that simply is not the case, as other variables come into play, such as genetics, lifestyle, and of course, stress. I see plenty of people who have great skin and imperfect diets, and vice versa. I also see people who lead so-called healthy lives—they eat right, exercise, and generally take good care of themselves—but who are still plagued by premature aging, acne, and troubling skin conditions.

Nutritional medicine is a rapidly growing area of research that will continue to gain momentum as we learn more and more about the connections between nutrition and health—not just in relation to skin health, but all kinds of health concerns. In fact, the link between nutrition and diseases like obesity, diabetes, cancer, and cardiovascular disease are well documented. I expect us to learn more and more about the powerful influences diet can have on our skin health and ability to slow down the inevitable decline we call *aging* and its appearance on our bodies. Because we know that oxidative stress, inflammation, and, to a lesser extent, genetics, are the chief agers in our bodies, and because they spur chronic conditions that wear us down physically, gaining the upper hand on these as best we can is key. And if diet can help this in any way, then we should be paying attention.

I also want to note that there is no single approach to optimizing health and beauty, and that diet alone is not the answer. As this program clearly demonstrates, the combination of proven skin-care techniques, relaxation therapies to dampen stress, exercise, restful sleep, and diet are all important and play a part in your looks on the inside *and* the outside. It would be impossible to say which of these factors is more important than the other. They all bear weight, and perhaps which one carries the most depends on the individual, especially as they relate to a person's genetics and other lifestyle choices. I will reiterate, however, that I do believe stress is an underlying theme in much of what we see today in the patterns of disease and aging in Western society. We may find, for example, that all this chatter about the Western diet being the ultimate villain in causing cancer, cardiovascular disease, and diobesity (the buzzword for obesity and diabetes) is like missing the forest for the trees. In other words, we may be wrapping our focus around diet so much that we forget to address the bigger, more omnipotent villain: stress. After all, even when it comes to diet, stress can take hold of us and affect what we choose to eat, how much we eat, and how our bodies respond accordingly. In essence, stress is at the top of this metaphorical food chain—tripping a cascade of events that can lead to thicker waistlines, dour moods, poor sleep, chronic inflammation and oxidative stress, and, as a result, an unhealthy body and appearance. You look as bad as you feel—sick and tired.

On the bright side, if stress is such an influential cast member in our world, and we can learn how to control it with the help of optimal diet choices, then we may be able to manage the balancing act so that we achieve peak health and beauty. And that's exactly what we're going to do. But first, let me sum up the main points to the diet-skin connection.

The Two Biggest Ways Diet Can Affect Your Looks

There's no doubt that the ritual of eating has a commanding role in our lives. Food is satisfying and soothing, as well as energizing and revving. What's more, there is something deeply cultural and spiritual about sitting down to eat and bringing a fork or spoon to the mouth with delight. What we put in our mouths says a lot about who we are, what we like, and how we live. Of course, with that comes the reality that what we eat helps determine how we look and feel, and whether or not we are overweight, underweight, poised to run a marathon, at risk for insulin resistance and diabetes, able to fight off illness quickly, or armed with an arsenal of weapons to stem the onset of age-related disease. Age-related diseases, mind you, that dictate the state of your physical looks, too.

Given what we currently know about this elusive diet-beauty connection, the following are two of the most important features.

Hormonal responses to nutrients. I don't think anyone can deny the food-mood connection. Throughout this book you are learning about myriad ways hormones can affect biochemical pathways as well as your psychology, which in turn influence physical health and beauty. When you are hungry, you feel and act hungry, scouring for your next source of energy to give you a boost both physically and mentally. You are likely cranky, too, caring more about getting something in your mouth, regardless of what that something is (although simple carbs sound delicious right about now). If you find a high-sugar item, your blood sugar will surge and, in response, insulin will rush out to escort sugar into cells where it can be used for energy and metabolism. The body will pump out lots of insulin when faced with lots of sugar so that there is no excess lingering in the blood.

This large insulin response can then trigger a dramatic drop in blood sugar—sometimes to levels that are even too low—in the hours after the food is eaten. When blood glucose levels fall, guess what: Your body senses stress and prompts a surge of those famous adrenal stress hormones adrenaline and cortisol. And, by now, you have a clear understanding about how cortisol ages you from the inside out.

Fat Fix

Studies show that more than 70 percent of those who undereat or overeat during a stressful period admit to snacking on foods that are nutrient poor. Fats and sugars seem to fit the bill during times of stress.

Preventing this roller-coater ride in your bloodstream that leads to a stress response is all about keeping those blood sugars balanced. This is accomplished by choosing complex carbohydrates that are high in fiber, lean proteins, and healthy fats, all of which foster a slow and steady digestion. It's like the difference between driving a car like a maniac through stop-and-go traffic (fast, slow, fast, slow) versus keeping the speedometer at a steady pace. The body, like your car, prefers the latter approach—much less wear and tear. In doing so, you will be able to avoid those crazy, bingeing moments when you feel so out of control.

The fact that food can trigger your stress-response system is significant. Numerous studies have shown that an overactive stress response is associated with overeating, changes in blood chemistry and hormones, and, in particular, a decrease in the amino acid tryptophan. Why is this important? Tryptophan is a necessary building block in the mood-regulating neurotransmitter called *serotonin.* As you know, low levels of serotonin are linked to depression (or simply a depressed mood), insomnia, anxiety, anger, and continued bingeing on sugary, fatty foods. All of this can then lead to weight gain, especially the most unhealthy kind of all, around the midlines and waistlines. Like a drug addict looking for his next hit, we want this serotonin when we attack the kitchen seeking sugary, nutrient-poor carbohydrates. Our brains release a short burst of serotonin when we eat simple sugars and carbohydrates; we feel good for a moment, but soon return to our low-serotonin state, and crash and burn. That's when we crave more sugar and simple carbohydrates in hopes of feeling that little high again . . . and the downward spiral continues.

One more thought I want to share before moving on. All too often people think of fat as something that is sedentary or dormant. Much to the contrary, fat is highly active, and can even generate its own messengers and chemicals, including hormones. Abdominal fat in particular has been the highlight of several studies. In 2005, researchers demonstrated that abdominal fat cells produce cortisol in large amounts. Fat cells can also release chemical messengers that promote inflammation. Japanese researchers have found that fat cells can generate free radicals that can then do damage throughout the body. They concluded that excess abdominal fat may bring on systemwide oxidative stress that has profound effects all over your body. Yes, that means your fat could be playing a secret role in your collagen breakdown. So the lesson is clear: Achieving and maintaining an ideal weight and a healthy muscle-to-fat ratio is important. You can do that using the diet guidelines in this chapter.

Hormonal responses to what you consume go much deeper than those I just described. But I just want you to have a general understanding of how this plays out in the body. It's a vicious cycle, too, as stressors in our lives have the potential to negatively persuade us to choose the wrong foods, which, in turn, influence our body's stress response system and ultimately, our appearance.

Food is medicine. All the tools our bodies need to function optimally and efficiently can be found in foods. We need food to live, to maintain the structure and function of our cells, and to support and fuel the systems that keep us going strong—from our immune system to our digestive, respiratory, circulatory, and so on. However, some foods can lack nutrients we need, and when we perpetually consume nutrient-poor foods and beverages that are filled with harmful impersonators such as hydrogenated trans fats, saturated fats, and refined sugars, topped with preservatives, additives, and artificial flavors and colors, we set ourselves up for downgrading our health.

This happens because our bodies lose the capacity to self-heal efficiently as inflammation pathways take over and our natural sources of antioxidants are used up. In addition, the stress we bear can rapidly deplete our bodies' supply of desperately needed nutrients to the point we become deficient in a few choice ones pivotal to our natural defense mechanisms, such as magnesium, zinc, and selenium. Without ample supplies nearby and continual replenishment, the

Fat Ain't Foolish

Just when you thought fat was as stationary and inactive as a hibernating bear, think again: It can secrete hormones and chemical messengers that will do exactly what you don't want, which is telling your body to stay fat and break down beauty-enhancing collagen.

flames of aging, inflammation, and free-radical mayhem hit high marks. And, when the stress simmers over long periods of time—maybe forever—the entire waterfall effect among hormones, inflammatory chemicals, and free radicals sets the stage for accelerated and potentially irreversible aging.

There is nothing wrong with eating, say, fast food and refined sugar, in moderation; it is the chronic abuse of these nutrient-poor foods that is a problem. I'm not the first to hawk the idea of everything in moderation, but it's really true that moderation is key to establishing a successful relationship with food and eating. I also understand the need for certain comfort foods and sugar on occasion. They make us feel good, can lift a bad mood, and plain and simple be a form of stress relief. In that regard, sugar can be medicine, too! The secret is to combine sugar with other ingredients, so it doesn't promote body chaos and send you through swinging highs and lows. If you eat sugar after a meal rich in lean proteins, healthy fats, and complex carbs, or eat sugar alongside these types of hormone-friendly foods, it won't incite such a huge insulin response as it would on its own.

the short story on inflammation and uv rays

We'll get to the buffet in a moment, but first we need to make a detour into the lab and tangle with two skin enemies in the context of food: inflammation and the sun's ultraviolet light.

First, let's explore more about inflammation, a term that you've no doubt read numerous times since beginning this book. It's practically a celebrity on its own, and given its exposure in the media lately, you already may be familiar with it. At this writing, a Google search on inflammation turns up about 27.8 *million* hits, and there will be many more by the time this book is in your hands. Researchers are hot on inflammation's trail because, as I just mentioned, it helps to explain how killers like heart disease, diabetes, and cancer gain a foothold in our bodies. We are now just beginning to make scientific links between certain kinds of inflammation in the body and the most pernicious degenerative diseases today, including Alzheimer's, autoimmune diseases, and an accelerated aging process in general. Volumes of international research clearly indicate that it's tied to virtually all chronic conditions.

Inflammation is supposed to be a good thing, a way for the body to fend off harmful bacteria, viruses, and other elements that could be toxic to us. On a most basic level, we're all familiar with the kind of inflammation that accompanies cuts and bruises—pain, swelling, heat, and redness. Allergies and arthritis are also forms of inflammation. When injured tissue becomes inflamed, the body reacts by calling in the immune-system troops to quell the heat and injury. Even the redness and swelling around an acne lesion is low-grade inflammation in action.

However, chronic inflammation acts like a smoldering wildfire in our bodies. When inflammation goes awry, it can disrupt the immune system and trip chronic problems or disease. The scary-sneaky part about inflammation is that it can be going on inside us at a deep level without us really knowing it because we can't necessarily *feel* it. Eventually, you do have to take note of it when it builds up over time and results in an ailment or disease, from simple skin rashes and persistent acne to more serious problems like heart disease and cancer.

A Fiery Fact

Inflammation creates an imbalance in the body that can stimulate negative effects not only on your skin, but in your entire body.

What fuels the endless burn of chronic inflammation? Oxidative stress, or free-radical damage that can cause wrinkles and cancer. Because free radicals steal electrons from other molecules, rendering those molecules handicapped and damaged, they both trigger inflammation and are created by it.

The sun's UV light also generates an army of free radicals. It's estimated that *half* of the sun's skin damage is caused by them. Inflammation and UV assaults are like a one-two punch to your skin because its major components—fats, proteins, and DNA—are favorite free-radical targets. The end result is, yes, skin aging: Collagen breaks down, abnormal elastin increases, moisture is lost, wrinkles accumulate, and skin cancer may start brewing, too.

What you eat can help turn down the burn and protect skin from UV damage. Though diet alone can't turn back chronological time, it may be able to slow the biological clock. Our innate defense system against free radicals and inflammation is partially dependent on dietary sources of antioxidants. Yes, your body's cells can manufacture antioxidants, but they still require certain raw materials in the form of dietary nutrients to create them and make them useful. Your triple reward: Not just your skin but also your body and mind will benefit.

End of detour, on to the beauty buffet. We've picked up a plate; let's start filling it.

Colorful Fact

The reason fruits and veggies come in such bright colors are antioxidants, many of which are actually colorful pigments. For instance, beta-carotene gives sweet potatoes, cantaloupe, and carrots their orangey hue, and lycopene makes tomatoes and watermelon red. Antioxidants don't just make plants pretty colors; these pigments help fend off environmental attacks from ultraviolet radiation, bugs, fungus, and more. Human skin has its own supplies of many of these nutrients, but they get depleted in fighting off free radicals. That's why you need to replenish by eating lots of jewel-colored fruits and vegetables.

the beauty buffet

I know what you're asking: What do I *eat*? Forget about what you *can't* eat for now (FYI: There are no off-limits foods unless you are allergic), and focus on all that's good for you and your skin. Diet books often use the so-called plate method to show readers how to create a healthy plate, and that's what we're going to do here. It's as easy as 1-2-3-4. The following is an example of what a plate should look like for beautiful skin.

First, Pile on the Veggies and Fruits

Grab enough to fill fully half your plate, not a measly corner or two (the daily goal: nine—yes, *nine*—half-cup servings). Fruits and veggies are brimming with antioxidants, vitamins, minerals, and phytochemicals, which are other protective plant substances known to help humans, too. All of these act like the dietary highway patrol, pulling over speeding free radicals and suspending their licenses to create havoc. How? Eating lots of veggies and fruits helps replenish our natural antioxidant stores, protecting sun-exposed skin against wrinkling and even skin cancer.

The abundant vitamin C in these foods may be particularly beneficial. Vitamin C is involved in the production of collagen, and the skin of women whose diets are rich in C is the least likely to have signs of aging, like thinning, dryness, and wrinkles. The benefits don't happen overnight—you need to keep topping up the tank with these superfuels. So be sure to eat your greens . . . and reds, purples, orange/yellows. In fact, go for the whole rainbow; mixing colors throughout the week will ensure you get the variety you need.

By the way, organic fruits and veggies usually cost more but are worth the price. Organically grown produce appears to churn out higher levels of antioxidants as well as containing far fewer pesticides than the regular (conventionally grown) stuff. Recent test case: Organic tomatoes turn out to have *twice* the antioxidant flavonols as conventionally grown ones.

Chew Up Fat with Vitamin C?

Vitamin C is more than an antioxidant. It's essential to your body's breakdown and utilization of food, and your body can neither manufacture it on its own nor store it, which means that you need to get a constant supply of vitamin C from food sources, or from supplementation. In the last twenty-five years, the level of vitamin C deficiency in our population has increased, partly due to our processed food supplies that are low on the nutrient meter. Some studies are now showing that vitamin C may also give your metabolism a boost, increasing your fat-burning capacity by 30 percent! Researchers have demonstrated that vitamin C can reduce age-related weight gain, and that too little vitamin C in the blood correlates with increased body fat and wider waistlines.

Second, Garnish Your Fruits and Veggies with Nuts, Seeds, or a Bit of Olive-Oil-Based Dressing

Nuts and seeds are full of vitamin E, another off-the-charts antioxidant that, like C, is abundant in skin. Plus the sun depletes our stores of E, so if you live an outdoor life, you need to be vigilant about replacing it. Both E and C have been incorporated into a plethora of cosmetics, but they can act like fish out of water in topical formulas. Because they are so unstable and at the mercy of light and oxygen in the air, it's hard to be sure these antioxidants that you try to sink into your skin actually get to where they are needed. All the more reason to eat E- and C-rich foods.

Olive oil is also rich in antioxidants, but its real skin benefit appears to be its good fats (the monounsaturated kind). These healthy fats seem to help cells resist photoaging, which surfaces as wrinkling. Other foods that may help protect sun-exposed skin from wrinkles include vegetables and legumes—beans, lentils, and chickpeas.

Kitchen Switch

See if you can replace your butter and margarine with extra-virgin olive oil and canola oil for cooking. You can find sprays of these oils in the market for pan-frying, too. Also try switching from processed peanut butter to 100 percent pure, organic peanut butter (you should see nothing but nuts in the ingredients).

Third, Fill a Quarter of Your Plate with Lean Protein

Every cell in your body needs protein to thrive but what else arrives with that protein can make a big skin and health difference. What you want: healthy fats and certain skin-essential minerals and vitamins. What you don't: aging fats, meaning the saturated fats found in steak and other red meats, as well as in fat-oozing creamy cheeses and other full-fat dairy foods. They don't do any part of your body good. So, when you think skin and protein, think fish, white meat poultry, tofu, and legumes.

- Choose wild salmon or mackerel for their healthy omega-3 fatty acids—yup, these fats fight inflammation and may help protect against sunburn.
- Also choose tuna and salmon, as well as shellfish (lobster, clams, and crabs) for their selenium, which partners with vitamin E to keep your birthday suit smooth and unwrinkled.
- Eat dark leafy greens like spinach and orange ones like carrots; they're a quick way to get your daily vitamin A, which helps revitalize skin's surface by increasing cell turnover. (Vitamin A's skin rub-on version, tretinoin, is by far the best wrinkle fighter around.)
- And don't forget beans, chickpeas, lentils, and other protein-filled legumes. Along with poultry and some fortified cereals, they supply skin with zinc, which is essential for the antioxidant activity and cell division. One of the first signs that zinc is in short supply is troubled skin. Shortfalls of the mineral are linked to eczema and slow wound healing.

Lean proteins afford you numerous benefits that show up in your skin. They are, after all, the building blocks of life, helping you to maintain the natural structures and functions of your body. Some underappreciated tasks of proteins: They are responsible for repairing and rebuilding muscle tissues (including vulnerable tissues in the skin!), they grow hair and nails, they create enzymes and hormones (including ones that belong in the chain of events leading to vibrant skin), and they maintain the health of your internal organs and blood. Can't pull away from the table soon enough? Eat more protein because it helps satisfy you. And a good source of protein will also help you to recover from a workout so that you're ready to go again the next day.

Forget Fat-free

Don't omit fats entirely, especially the healthy ones like monounsaturated olive oil. Healthy fats help fat-soluble vitamins such as A, D, E, and K move around the body, create sex hormones, lower LDL (bad) cholesterol while boosting HLD (good) cholesterol, and contribute to the health of skin, eyes, nails, and hair.

Fourth, Fill That Last Quarter of Your Plate with Whole Grains

Say goodbye to refined carbs and white bread. There is nothing wondrous about Wonder Bread. You've heard about the new rule by now: Stick to whole grains like whole-wheat pasta and couscous, brown rice, barley, oatmeal, and bulgur. These and less familiar but equally delicious whole grains, such as quinoa and amaranth, are filled with skin-helping, stress-hampering ingredients. Among them:

- Antioxidants, including vitamin E, and the antioxidant helpers selenium and zinc
- A smidge of healthy fatty acids, including skin-smoothing linoleic acid
- Calming complex carbs (another serotonin source)

In addition, unlike highly processed simple carbs (white rice, white pasta, white-flour anything), which trigger sharp, unhealthy blood-sugar spikes that can add to physical stress, complex whole-grain carbs are *full* of fiber. That means they are absorbed slowly, which keeps blood sugar steady, so that your energy is less likely to slump. Fiber, in this regard, helps keep your metabolism humming. You can also think of whole grains as the carbs that keep you sane. With steady blood-sugar levels come steady moods. And we all can agree that steady moods make for less stress. We are much less likely to attack the kitchen at full throttle for a high-fat, high-sugar fix.

Sound Familiar?

One in four Americans turns to food help alleviate stress. I'm surprised it's not more.

How to nix the fix. It may take time to wean yourself from refined sugars, unhealthy carbs, and processed foods, especially if you've been eating them regularly for years. It helps to clean out your kitchen and throw away anything that has the following words in its ingredients: enriched and bleached flour, high-fructose corn syrup, or hydrogenated and partially hydrogenated oils.

And, while you're at it, toss anything with the word *sugar* in the first five ingredients, unless it's a dessert item that you want to keep for an occasional splurge!

The Stress-Fighting Stars: Magnesium and Zinc

As your freak-out level rises, your need for magnesium jumps, too. Magnesium reduces an overactive stress-response system, and inadequate amounts can increase substance P—that nervous system chemical that promotes pain and is known to be involved in the stress-response pathway in the skin. (Trivia: the *P* actually stands for *powder;* when isolated for the first time from horse intestine in the 1930s, it was in powder form.) Be sure you're getting at least 400 mg a day—most people don't—from a variety of magnesium-rich foods, such as soy milk, black beans, poultry, halibut, and chard.

Unlike media stars vitamin C, calcium, and iron, zinc doesn't get a lot of ink. Besides, most nutritional sources say you're probably getting enough to keep your skin glowing. Enough, that is, unless you're:

- vegetarian
- breastfeeding
- cutting back on cholesterol
- eating a lot of processed foods
- taking calcium supplements
- suffering from IBS (irritable bowel syndrome)
- trying to lose weight
- taking iron supplements

That adds up to a lot of itchy, flaky skin complaints that could be linked to a lack of zinc. Zinc is one of those workhorse nutrients that's involved in almost every biochemical reaction in your body, but it's especially important for skin cell renewal. Zinc isn't hard to find—shellfish, lean ham, beef, and lamb are full of it (which is why vegetarians need to work a bit harder to get enough). As the preceding list shows, it's easy to throw off zinc levels. A lot of things can either drain the body's supplies (breastfeeding) or interfere with zinc's absorption (almost everything else; calcium supplements alone can cut it in half). How much zinc do you need, and how can you get enough to keep your skin's RealAge young? The recommended daily value is 15 mg, the amount in most multivitamins. Aim to get a little more, especially if you're dealing with anything on the list. Good sources include:

Oysters. They're the all-stars; depending on the type, they can run from 16 mg per half dozen to 40 mg or more, but they are hardly a staple food.

Fortified breakfast cereals. They can be terrific; for instance, a cup of Cheerios has 15 mg. Just be sure your cereal doesn't have more sugar than zinc.

Several of the following every day. Meat, chickpeas, lentils, dairy foods, and nuts. With a good mix of these, it's easy to get your daily dose, but don't go overboard. Getting more than the upper limit of 40 mg can cause heart-healthy good HDL cholesterol to plummet and throw off your immune system. Topically speaking, you can also use a zinc cream on dry skin patches. Diaper rash creams, such as Vusion, work well, and come in handy during those winter months. The zinc oxide makes a terrific barrier against moisture loss and protects skin from external irritants.

what to drink at the beauty bar

Personally, I start with water. Dehydration looks and feels lousy: It saps skin and triggers fatigue. Fill your glass regularly and add a squeeze of lemon or orange if you like. Listen to your thirst signals; you don't have to check off eight full glasses of pure water a day. This old recommendation was busted earlier this year when two kidney experts had a scientific review published in the *Journal of the American Society of Nephrology*. In it, they show there's no clear-cut scientific rationale for the average healthy individual to drink eight glasses of water or more a day. Remember, too, that you get water through a variety of sources like fruits, vegetables, and teas.

I get most of my water by drinking tea. I'm crazy about tea. I always have been, but now there are powerful reasons to drink it. Researchers have learned that all true teas—that is, those that come from the *Camellia sinensis* plant, which includes black, green, white, and oolong—have two dazzling skin benefits. They prevent *photoaging* (wrinkling) and fight skin cancer. Green tea has an edge because it has the highest levels of a powerful antioxidant known as *epigallocatechin-3-gallate* (EGCG), which has a lion-tamer effect on tumor cells. EGCG can suppress the inflammatory chemicals that are directly involved in skin reactions, including acne. Green tea has more antioxidants than black, but both help squelch free radicals and subdue inflammation. Aim for four to six cups of tea per day.

Before noon is my black-tea time, then I have green tea at lunch and sip it during afternoon breaks in the office, because the bit of caffeine perks me up. Aromatic jasmine tea is my favorite fragranced tea. When I don't want the buzz, such as after dinner, I brew hojicha green tea (available at www.adagio.com and www.itoen.com). The roasting process that turns this green tea a brownish color also lowers its caffeine content. If you're caffeine sensitive, just choose decaf tea—its health pluses don't seem to be affected by the decaf process—or put your cup away at least three hours before heading to bed. Pregnant and breast-feeding women may also want to stick to decaf teas.

The only downside to drinking lots of tea is that it stains your teeth because it's high in tannins. Mixing a tiny bit of baking soda into your toothpaste helps keep staining to a minimum between dental cleanings.

Tea versus Stress

Any warm drink is a super stress soother, and curling up with a cup of aromatic jasmine tea can make the whole day go away. But with tea, it's not just the warmth at work. Skin-friendly tea also has two magic antistress ingredients: *L-theanine,* an amino acid that produces a relaxed but alert frame of mind, and *catechins,* antioxidants that, among other things, lower *corticosterone,* a stress hormone.

Another way to drink your antioxidants is via dark cocoa, which is rich in a particularly potent group of flavonols. In fact, cocoa has two to three times the antioxidants of green tea and four to five times more than black tea but, unfortunately, many more calories. Still, it is *really* good for skin: In a recent study, a daily dose of cocoa for just six weeks made skin smoother, better hydrated, and less sun sensitive, and twelve weeks did even more. It wasn't just the flavonols; the dark cocoa boosted nourishing circulation to the skin.

To tap cocoa's skin powers, skip cocoa mixes, which don't have the same flavonol levels, and go for the real thing: dark, unadulterated cocoa powder that contains 70 percent or more cacao. Scharffen Berger natural cocoa powder and Ghirardelli unsweetened cocoa are two examples of brands that pass the test; others include Droste, Fauchon, and Jacques Torres. Here is my husband Harry's hot chocolate recipe.

Harry's Super-Simple Healthy Hot Cocoa

The only secret to this recipe is patience: Heat it s-l-o-w-l-y.

The flavor will be better and the slow heat will release more antioxidants.

1 ½ teaspoons unsweetened cocoa powder with 70% or more cacao

2 teaspoons sugar

Pinch of salt

1 cup skim or low-fat milk

Combine all ingredients in a saucepan and heat slowly, stirring frequently, until it's just beginning to steam. Do not boil. Pour into a mug and enjoy.

Don't stop with tea and cocoa. Savor four ounces of red wine for its *resveratrol*—an antioxidant and anti-inflammatory that's showing a lot of promise as a protector against UVB damage. One glass a day is the healthy limit for women, up to two for men. I like to have mine before dinner instead of a cocktail. Or pass up the vino and down some pomegranate juice (for sparkle and more H_2O, mix it with bubbly water and serve in a wine glass). It's so rich in antioxidants that it's like liquid gold for your skin and body.

eight soothing foods to calm you down fast

Nutritionists and diet gurus know that the two rules to healthy eating and slimmer waistlines are: Always eat a nutritious breakfast within an hour of rising, and eat every three to four hours thereafter. Of course, *what* you eat is also important, and can go a long way toward remedying, and preventing, sags and slumps during your day. Avoiding that sensation of being off-the-charts ravenous will help you to fight mental fatigue and subzero energy. It will also help you to make better food choices at your next meal or snack.

When your to-do list has you running on coffee and doughnuts, it's probably time to rethink more than just your diet. Start by reorganizing by priority: What must be done today? What can wait a day or two? A week? Forever? Then ask for help. At home, get family members to kick in with chores and errands, which can include cooking, tidying up the kitchen, and emptying the dishwasher. For big projects, tap a best friend or two. At work, brush up your delegation skills or ask a coworker to pitch in and promise to return the favor. And reach for foods that *really* fight stress, like these seven wonders of the high-wired world. (Note: for another list of excellent food ideas, see Appendix B: Seven Foods That Fight Slumps.)

Berries, Any Berries

Blackberries, strawberries, cranberries, raspberries, blueberries. They're not just delicious; they're among fifty foods in the American diet with the highest levels of antioxidants, which is why they're great at countering the skin-damaging free radicals generated by stress. Eat them one by one (like healthy M&Ms) when the pressure is on. If you're a jaw clencher, try rolling a frozen berry around in your mouth. And then another, and another.

Guacamole

If you're craving something creamy, look no further. Avocados are loaded with B vitamins, which stress quickly depletes and which your body needs to maintain nerves and brain cells. Their creaminess comes from healthy monounsaturated fats—the same kind that makes olive oil good for your skin. Scoop up the stuff with whole-grain baked chips or raw veggies. If you're watching calories, dip instead of scoop: Two tablespoons have about fifty-five calories.

Nuts

Almost all nuts are good sources of vitamins B and E, plus selenium and zinc, but some have a more than others. To get the biggest nutritional bang for your buck, mix them up: Just an ounce will help replace those stress-depleted Bs (walnuts); give you a whopping amount of selenium and zinc (Brazil nuts), which are also drained by high anxiety; boost your vitamin E (almonds), which helps fight cellular damage linked to chronic stress; and may even lower your blood pressure by helping your arteries relax (pistachios). An ounce of nuts is about a small handful, such as twenty-three almonds. Don't overdo nuts, because they are high in calories. Buy nuts in the shell and think of it as multitasking: With every squeeze of the nutcracker, you're releasing a little bit of tension.

Oranges

People who take a 1,000 mg of vitamin C before giving a speech have lower levels of cortisol and better-behaved blood pressure than those who don't. So lean back, take a deep breath, and concentrate on peeling a big, juicy orange. The five-minute mindfulness break will steady your brain cells and you'll get a bunch of C as well. Just don't fastidiously remove all the zest: Protective phytochemicals are usually concentrated in the skins of fruits.

Asparagus

Each tender stalk is a source of *folate*, a B vitamin that appears to be essential for mood and proper nerve function in the brain. Dip the stalks in yogurt for a hit of calcium with each bite.

Salmon and Other Fatty Fish

The omega-3 fatty acid in salmon, called docosahexaenoic acid or DHA, isn't just good for your skin. Studies show people who eat ample amounts of DHA have a much lower incidence of depression, aggressiveness, and hostility. So, this healthy fish may even help road rage! Some people report improvements in mood within days or even hours of eating omega-3-rich meals.

Q: I hate salmon with a passion (I've tried all types—Atlantic, wild, smoked, poached, etc.), and yet every doctor seems to hawk its health benefits to the point at which I feel I should force-feed myself. Should I?

A: Of course not! Yes, salmon is overly touted as a superfood because it imparts lots of healthy (omega-3) fats and is a rich source of proteins, but it's not the only place to get these ingredients. Eating should be an enjoyable, delectable experience, so forget trying to love salmon and, instead, seek alternatives that are equally superb. Examples include other cold-water fish, such as Alaskan halibut, sardines, herring, trout, sea bass, oysters, and clams. If you dislike fish in general, omega-3 fatty supplements are great to take daily. Another substitute food for fish is vegetarian-fed eggs, which contain the same fish oil found in marine sources of this terrific fatty acid.

Q: How concerned should I be about polluted, mercury-laden fish?

A: Enough to opt for wild, organic varieties whenever you can. Don't stress out about this or avoid fish entirely. The pros of eating fish outweigh the cons. Most markets carry wild varieties of fish, and if you go to the canned fish section of the supermarket, you'll find canned Alaskan salmon, which is always wild.

It's not surprising that omega-3s and brain health go hand in hand. About two-thirds of your brain is composed of fats. When you digest the fat in your food, it's broken down into fatty acid molecules of various lengths. Your brain then uses these for raw materials to assemble the special types of fat it incorporates into its cell membranes. The protective sheath that covers communicating neurons, for instance, is composed of 30 percent protein and 70 percent fat.

This is why it's very important that we get essential fatty acids, otherwise known as the family of omega-3s and 6s, which come from foods like fish, avocado, almonds, walnuts, flax seeds, and olives, on a daily basis. They are essential because your body can't manufacture them on its own. The reason salmon is called *brain food* is that it contains this high-quality fat. (All omega-

3s have numerous health benefits, but those that are found in fish are known as *long-chain omega-3s*, which researchers suspect may protect against coronary heart disease.) When we start eating saturated, trans, and hydrogenated fats, we aren't nourishing our brains; we're filling the fat cells that become weight elsewhere—on our hips, thighs, upper backs, and behind our arms. Trans fatty acids in particular, found in foods like french fries, margarine, potato chips, and anything else with partially hydrogenated oil, have been shown to disrupt communication in your brain.

Aim for at least two helpings a week of fatty fish, such as salmon, herring, mackerel, or sardines.

Spinach

Spinach and other happy greens (the dark, leafy ones) contain *folate*, that B vitamin essential to a good mood. Two cups of cooked spinach gives you the 400 micrograms of folate recommended to pick up your mood.

Dark Chocolate

No one knows for sure why we crave chocolate. It could be one of its hundreds of compounds, including caffeine, sugar, fat, *anandamide* (a feel-good brain chemical associated with states of bliss and delight), or *phenylethylamine* (another chemical that triggers feelings similar to falling in love), or simply the melt-in-your-mouth creamy texture. What we do know is that the antioxidant flavonols in dark chocolate (check labels; you want 70 percent or more cacao) help keep blood pressure steady and your mind sharp. They also may help counter cellular damage caused by stress. Try this when you need a mental lift: Microwave eight ounces of vanilla almond milk on medium for one minute, then stir in an ounce of dark chocolate till it melts (heat triggers antioxidant release). Delish. Just show a little restraint; chocolate packs a lot of calories.

Q. I barely have time to eat, much less focus on good skin foods. Aren't there some tricks for getting more healthy-skin nutrients into my diet?

A. Sometimes eating more fruits and vegetables seems as challenging as going out to the fields to pick our own corn, but it doesn't have to be that way. Here are some fast, fresh ways to get more of nature's good stuff into your body.

Fruit-and-Veggie Smoothies! They don't actually *taste* like veggies. Put this concoction in your blender: Lots of frozen berries (any kind), a splash of fruit juice or skim milk, and some of those vegetables you know you're missing—broccoli, cauliflower, beans, Brussels sprouts, whatever. The taste of the berries will overpower that of the vegetables, and you'll have a sweet treat that's packed with nutrient power.

Fruit Fries. Be religious about this. Whenever you're at a restaurant that offers french fries as a side dish, ask for fresh fruit instead. Don't let the waitstaff change your mind. Do the same thing at breakfast: fruit instead of bacon, sausage, or home fries.

Chop and Rock. Keep your cutting board handy at all times. Having an omelet or scrambled eggs? Toss in some chopped vegetables. Making a sandwich? Add a layer of chopped vegetables. Putting together a bowl of tuna, chicken, or salmon salad? Mix in some corn, chopped celery, onions, or dried cherries. No veggies in the bin? Keep chopped frozen veggies on hand and nuke a fistful in the microwave, or pour frozen ones directly into simmering soups, stews, and oven-ready casseroles (just up the cooking time by a few minutes).

Salad Bar Frenzy. Stop walking past the cafeteria salad bar and heading for the grill, no matter how good the burgers smell. Then, make like an artist: Assemble a palate of colors—reds, purples, greens, oranges, the works. It's a veritable smorgasbord of phytochemicals, fiber, and antioxidants. Each hue gives you a different piece of the nutritional puzzle. Add a few nuts or seeds and a drizzle of olive oil—all good fats—and you're golden.

Chicken Soup That *Really* Makes You Feel Better. Your mom was always a big chicken-soup promoter. Take it to the next level by loading yours up with different colored vegetables, just like a salad. It'll help your cold, too.

Pasta Plant Puree. A dish of whole-wheat pasta can get a big nutrient boost from tomato sauce made with pureed vegetables, which act as a nice thickener, too. Mmmm.

Grilling's Not Just for Meat. It's way easier to grill vegetables than a steak. Try kabobs made of peppers, zucchini, squash, tomatoes, or anything you have a hankering for. Brush with olive oil, sprinkle with herbs, and dig in.

Fruit, Not Cookies. For dessert, bake, microwave, or sauté a combination of apples, peaches, and plums tossed with cinnamon. Or, if you want an easy sweet fix, top angel food cake with strawberries and blueberries.

---

foods to skimp on or avoid

There are a couple of good-skin reasons to go easy on particular foods, specifically:

- red and processed meats
- full-fat milk and dairy products
- soft drinks (diet and regular)
- cakes and pastries

Solid research has linked diets high in these foods to sun-triggered wrinkling and even skin cancer. First, a ten-year Australian study found that people who habitually eat a meat-and-fat-rich diet develop more skin cancer than those whose meals are full of veggies and fruit. Other studies linked sun damage and wrinkling to meat, fats, sweets, and sugar.

On the other hand, wrinkle-*discouraging* diets have, no big surprise here, centered around not only fruits and veggies but the other nutritional heroes:

beans, olive oil, nuts, whole-grain breads, and tea. You don't have to be a health nut or tea-leaf reader to deduce that cutting back on fatty, sugary, and/or highly processed foods and replacing them all with a plant-rich diet likely has skin benefits.

Can Sugar Really Cause Wrinkles?

Earlier, I mentioned a process called *glycation* that involves sugar's alleged role in skin aging. Glycation is another buzzword of late in beauty-and health-circles. Briefly, it's a reaction that occurs when sugar molecules bond with fats or proteins. It happens when, for instance, food manufacturers add sugar to french fries to turn them a dark honey color. It also can happen in your body: Sugar interacts with protein in your cells, causing inflammation, a surge in free radicals, and molecules aptly tagged AGEs. Researchers have linked AGEs to rigid arteries, wrinkles, gummed-up nerves, and other outcomes nobody wants.

The more sugar scientists feed lab animals, the older the animals' skin becomes—it literally ages, becoming less elastic and soft. Most of this research, however, has been done on diabetic animals whose sugar-metabolizing systems are not functioning normally. The jury is still out on exactly how glycation operates in a healthy human being with a fully functioning metabolism. It's not fair to state plainly that "sugar causes wrinkles," because that's too much of a stretch, and there are multiple layers of metabolic pathways and biological factors at work here.

That said, I don't want you to miss the other message. Considering the sugary state of the American diet (each of us eats about 100 pounds of added sugar per year), we would do well to manage our sugar intake, so we can avoid the potential consequences such as type 2 (non-insulin-dependent) diabetes and the ravages of that disease, which can, as we are seeing now in society and in the lab, prematurely age you. The good news is glycation has been reversed in diabetics simply by bringing high blood sugar down to normal. And diabetes has also been reversed in people who gain control of their blood sugar and lose excess weight. Remember: balance, balance, balance.

how the flintstones can change your life

Almost all women—93 percent, to be precise—occasionally skip meals or eat a bowl of Cheerios for dinner. And if you're stressed? Well, you may gravitate toward a feast of fast food, or you may lose your appetite entirely and try going to bed high on adrenaline. Popping a daily multivitamin/mineral is a smart way to help fill in what may be missing in your diet, not to mention what stress burns up. Taking a multi is also cheaper than buying a bunch of individual nutrients. Look for a brand that:

- Has 100 percent of the daily value (DV) for most nutrients (however, know that some nutrients—calcium, for instance—are are too big to cram into a single pill);
- Takes your age into account. For example, many menstruating women need extra iron; however, after menopause, they usually require less iron but more B_{12}.

I've been taking chewable vitamins since I was a kid. When I became pregnant, I was nearly paralyzed by nausea and couldn't stomach the prenatal vitamins. So, I went to the drugstore, compared labels, and had one of those *aha* moments: I discovered that except for iron, folate, and calcium, I could get what I needed in Flintstones Complete. I took extra folate and calcium and ate more red meat to get the iron, which is what I think was making me sick in supplement form. Ever since, I've been chewing a tablet a day, which contains the recommended dose for adults and children over four.

Go ahead and take any brand-name multi, no fancy/expensive formulas needed. It's a good backstop for your healthy diet, though not a foundation. That said, there are a few individual nutrients that I recommend taking as well, because it's impossible to pack enough of them into one multi and because it's often difficult to get enough of them in food alone. While it's not clear whether they'll benefit your skin, they're good for all of you, and if they do even one nice thing for your skin, cool.

- **Crank up the calcium.** Okay, so it's not a skin mineral. It does, however, support your body's scaffolding (bones) so you're not just a shapeless, skin-covered blob. If you don't routinely eat three daily servings of calcium-rich foods (say, fat-free milk, ricotta, and yogurt), take a supplement. Calcium citrate is the most absorbable; avoid dolomite, bone meal, colloidal calcium, or oyster shells, which are often contaminated with toxic metals.

- **Add some D.** Many calcium supplements include D (to help absorption); buy the combo. D is called the sunshine vitamin because it's manufactured in the skin whenever you get about fifteen minutes of sunlight. If you're slathering on sunscreens (as you should) and/or you're dark skinned or live in the northern half of the country, it's surprisingly easy to run low on D. Plus many researchers now suspect the daily value (DV) for this vitamin is too low and recommend at least 1,000 IU (international units) a day, not the currently recommended 400 IU. Not coincidentally, a lack of D appears linked to low moods and mental fogginess. Make sure you take vitamin D_3, the kind your body makes.

- **Finally, boost your omega-3s.** Most of us consume far too many omega-6 fats, thanks to all the processed foods we eat, and way too few omega-3s, especially a type called *docosahexaenoic acid* (DHA). That imbalance appears to contribute to depression. For help in fighting gloom, try taking one to two grams daily of a fish oil supplement that includes both DHA and *eicosapentaenoic acid* (EPA), the two types of omega-3s most readily used by the body. The only side effect may be some fishy-tasting burping (if that happens, try an algae-based DHA supplement). Possible bonus: a bit of added protection against sunburn and sun-induced DNA damage. One caveat: If you're injured or planning to have surgery, be sure to let your doctor know that you are taking omega-3, because it is a blood thinner.

The Truth about Vitamin C and E Supplements and Skin Vitamins

What about individual nutrients or special skin-health formulas that claim to improve skin? These grab-bag concoctions, which are mostly a mix of antioxidants, are hugely popular. However, there's minimal proof of payoff, at least right now. Oodles of isolated antioxidants like vitamins C and E and phytochemicals like those found in green tea have been dazzling in the test tube. When fed to lab animals, they have been marvelous at protecting against sun damage, wrinkles, and cancer; making skin softer, moister, and smoother; and halting inflammation and signs of aging. Those effects almost disappear when single-nutrient pills are tested in people. Green tea polyphenol pills, for example, protect mice skin from UV damage and skin cancer but do *nada* for human skin. In a topical form, however, green tea is anti-inflammatory and photoprotective.

In fact, studies of isolated antioxidant pills in humans have overall been not only disappointing but actually worrisome. Disappointing because the supplements haven't staved off health trouble. Worrisome because studies have shown that people with various diseases, from heart problems to liver ailments, who took vitamins A, E, and/or beta-carotene supplements, either to try and stop the disease or keep it from coming back, had a greater risk of dying than those who didn't.

Punch line: The more research we do on antioxidants, the more it looks like they work best in our bodies when they are consumed with other vitamins, minerals, and probably other components we haven't even discovered yet. All of the antioxidant nutrients you need come packaged together whenever you eat a stalk of broccoli or a juicy plum or a slice of multigrain walnut-raisin bread. Put simply: Eat whole foods.

the bottom line

My final word on food and skin is the same well-worn advice doctors have dished out for years: Eat a varied diet that's heavy on fruits, veggies, whole grains, legumes, nuts, and calcium-rich foods. This diet won't ever go out of style.

I bet you can remember rolling your eyes as a teenager, staring up at your mother on her invisible soapbox as she said the same thing. The minute you got to make your own decisions about food, you were sucking back a Coke and munching on Doritos without a care in the world. That may seem like eons ago, but the advice really hasn't changed. What has: the incentive. Because now you know that combining the right diet with a few simple supplements is one of the best things you can do for every inch of your skin.

8

special treatment

Acne and Other Skin Conditions

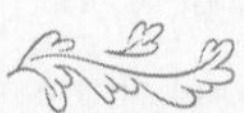

More than half of women (54 percent) over the age of twenty-five have acne. What happened? Weren't pimples supposed to go away forever when we graduated from high school . . . or, at least, college? Actually, one of the biggest sources of outrage in my office is women who can't believe they are getting pimples and wrinkles at the same time! It just doesn't seem fair. They think their bodies are going through an identity crisis, and the stress of worrying about the problem makes it all worse.

No one can say why these marks of adolescent and middle-aged skin are converging, but our love affair with the sun is probably saddling us with wrinkles far earlier than our moms or grandmas got them, and the stress of modern life is keeping acne in play. If acne were not such a problem, we would not be spending more than $100 million a year for various over-the-counter products. The overall cost of health care related to the treatment of acne exceeds $1 billion annually in the United States alone. That's a lot of money, and a lot of acne.

We now know a lot more about how to handle zits than when you were a teenager, so you can smooth and soothe your skin far faster than in the days when you were bemoaning breakouts to your study-hall buddies. This chapter is devoted to helping you address your acne, and it also includes insights on other common skin disorders. Acne gets most of the attention here, and for good reason: It's on the rise and affects at least 20 million adults; millions more probably never seek treatments.

Even though you may not be as emotional as you were at thirteen, acne may have a profound impact on your self-esteem and confidence. Your face is your most important feature, and it's usually the site where acne can be particularly troubling. We put our best foot forward, but we also try to put our best face forward when we present ourselves to the world, to our lovers, our bosses, our friends, our family, our coworkers, and ourselves in the mirror. It's no secret that our facial appearance is closely tied to body image. Let's not forget that dealing with acne can be an incredibly stressful and painful experience in more ways than one. The ultimate fallout from prolonged suffering from acne can be devastating as one becomes socially dysfunctional. The emotional toll, from depression, anger, frustration, anxiety, and embarrassment, can be overwhelming. This can then trickles into other aspects in life, including the ability to hold a job, have a career, relate well with others, and interact in healthy ways that support our well-being.

It is with all this in mind that we explore how to get a handle on acne, so that we don't let it control our lives. Before we get to clearing up your face, let's clear up some common misconceptions about acne.

truths and fictions

There are lots of myths around what triggers acne. At the top of most lists are oily skin and foods like chocolate and fried chicken. The origin of acne is more complicated than that and, as stated, there are plenty of people with oily skin and poor diets and perfectly clear skin. You can't necessarily blame last night's dinner or your oil-production level on your acne. At the root of virtually all acne is stress and inflammation; it's as simple as that.

Perception: I'm breaking out because I'm stressed.

Reality: You should know by now that stress turns on inflammatory pathways that result in breakouts. Genetics, menstruation, a new medication, the occasional irritating cosmetic can also contribute to acne, but stress is by far the most influential factor. Stressed or not, pimples appear when pores get clogged with skin cells that haven't sloughed off the way they should. What happens is the dead cells on your skin's surface get sticky, lining the follicle and clogging it up. Underneath is your sebum, where *P. acnes* bacteria show up for an oily meal, creating more inflammation. At the same time, immune system cells swarm in to deal with the mess.

Perception: I went on a chocolate binge yesterday; no wonder I woke up with a pimple.

Reality: Foods like chocolate, soda, pizza, potato chips, french fries—anything that seems bad or forbidden—usually get blamed for breakouts, but there's barely a lick of evidence showing any of them (or any food) produces pimples. I'm not convinced that all bad foods lead to pimples; in fact, I don't believe in any food being bad. I will take some of the current theories on the connection between diet and acne with a grain of salt until further research is done. Plus, a blemish usually takes longer to develop, so whatever you ate yesterday is irrelevant. Keep in mind that it's tempting to blame food because pimples make us feel out of control of our skin. If we decide chocolate is the culprit, we feel we can regain control if we stop eating it. If you swear you have a trigger food and you feel safer if you avoid it (and thus, it lowers your stress), by all means do. Personally, I wouldn't give up chocolate! I'd focus on treatment.

Perception: Maybe a day at the beach or a visit to the tanning parlor will get rid of my pimples.

Reality: The sun is deceptive. An hour on the beach today may dry up your acne a bit so that it looks better tomorrow, but a few days later, it's likely to be worse: more bumps, inflammation, and redness. Your skin reacts to the UV radiation by becoming inflamed; it reacts to the stress of those damaging rays with its own stress-response system, which you know by now can trigger acne and other troubling skin conditions. You may not see this for several days after sun exposure, and this delayed reaction can make you forget that it was the sun that caused all this to begin with. Save yourself the aggravation, and spare your skin the sun damage.

Perception: Moisturizer will just make breakouts worse.

Reality: Your skin still needs moisture. Even oily skin needs moisture. Acne meds are often very drying, so you may need more moisturizer, not less, when you are fighting breakouts. Otherwise, the overdryness may trigger inflammation, then you're back where you started: dealing with more acne. Just be sure to buy a formula that's *nonacnegenic* (look for the term *noncomedogenic*). For all practical purposes, if it's labeled oil-free, you're okay, too.

Perception: I never had acne as a teen, so it makes no sense that I have it now.

Reality: First, understand that adult acne is common and its causes are multifaceted. Not having zits as a teen doesn't confer lifelong protection. Hormones rise and fall, with pregnancy, during the various phases of menopause, and that's just one factor that can bring on acne. As women, we tend to take responsibility for everything. We think we cause our own stress, that it's up to us to deal with it, and, if we don't, it's our own fault. Same with acne: We think we're doing something to cause it. Not likely. Instead, focus on doing something to cure it and prevent it. Much smarter.

Q: What are the biggest myths about treating acne?

A: It's amazing how many strange ideas are out there.

- Many people put toothpaste on pimples because their grandmother told them it will dry the pimples out. It won't.
- Ditto for rubbing alcohol. People like the instantly cool feeling and they can see that it removes dirt. "Just look at the cotton ball," they say afterward. Well, yes, it removes surface dirt (so will washing your face) but it also strips off every bit of protective moisturizing oil from the surface, and getting rid of those oils won't get rid of the acne. That's another myth. It just makes your face painfully dry and flaky.
- Ditto for turpentine! Eek! Don't *ever* put turpentine on your skin!
- Ditto for a paste made out of baking soda and water—it's drying *and* abrasive. I do have a good use for baking soda and water, but it isn't treating pimples. It's cleaning jewelry. It's great for that. Ask any jeweler.
- There's one last big myth: that moisturizers make acne worse. The reality is that if skin gets too dry, and acne treatments can be very drying, *that* will make acne worse. In fact, people with somewhat oily skin may need to use moisturizer for the first time in their lives if they start to use acne treatments. Just be sure to buy a light, oil-free, *non-comedogenic* formula that doesn't contain glycolic acid or another exfolliant; they're too stressful to your skin if you're using an acne treatment.

anatomy of acne

At the heart of acne is simple inflammation of the *follicle*—the small oil-producing area and hair that make up a single pore. Recall from chapter 6 that the oil gland is called the *sebaceous gland* and secretes an oily substance called *sebum*. The oil-producing cells are continually replaced by new cells at the base of the gland, so sebum is actually a combo of both fat and old, dead cells. In a normal follicle, these old cells are brought up to the surface of the skin to shed via the hair shaft. Old cells lining the follicle will also fall from the wall and shed, too. The oil gland helps orchestrate this turnover by keeping the skin well lubricated, so those old cells can move up and out. Problems can arise if something goes wrong and the pores get clogged with gunk, from dead cells and sebum fats to excess *P. acnes* bacteria that normally reside in the follicle but in a controlled state.

stopping adult acne

A pimple at any age is disheartening, and women get them at every age. If you've never had to treat a pimple in your life, you're very lucky. (I certainly wasn't. I had raging acne as a teen that lasted until I went to college.) Most people, at one point or another, need some on-the-spot treatment. Fortunately, there are solutions for everyone.

The Number One Don't

No matter how tempting it is to squash, squeeze, or pick at pimples, don't. Why? Scarring, marks, and more inflammation. (You're getting something out, but you're also pushing junk in, exacerbating inflammation. You'll get a *new* pimple right next door in a few days.) Your nails are sharp and have bacteria under them, so you risk damaging skin's deeper layers and creating new pimples right next to the one you're picking. You can do *something*: Apply a warm compress on a blemish to loosen the thick oily plug of sebum. Then take two clean cotton swabs, place one on each side of the pimple, and apply gentle, even inward pressure. If something comes out, great; pat the spot dry and put on a treatment, such as your acne product. If not, leave it alone—it's not ready to budge.

Mild Acne

There are two really effective drugstore treatments for acne—benzoyl peroxide (BP) and salicylic acid—but they do different things and act in different ways. Benzoyl peroxide mainly kills *P. acnes,* the bacteria that can proliferate in a pore and causes acne, but it's quite drying and irritating. Salicylic acid is both an exfoliant—removing dead skin cells that can clog pores—and an anti-inflammatory. It's significantly less irritating, which is why I prefer salicylic acid.

If your skin is prone to dryness anyway, start with salicylic acid (a cream or lotion, not a wash) and give it two or three weeks to work. If that isn't enough, add benzoyl peroxide for a couple of weeks. If *that* combination isn't enough, don't start doubling or tripling products and treatments—your skin will overreact and get even worse. If you're still getting new breakouts, it's time to see a dermatologist. You need prescription-strength help.

When you're buying salicylic acid products, look for maximum strength, which is 2 percent. That's actually pretty mild. You can use salicylic acid products on your whole face, if you'd like; they'll act as an exfoliant and calm any redness. (Two other exfoliators, resorcinol and sulfur, have been used for years, but there isn't much evidence of their effectiveness.)

Benzoyl peroxide should usually be used as a spot treatment; it's too irritating to use all over your face (the exception is if you're using a mild BP wash when you cleanse your face). With BP, it doesn't matter whether you buy gels, pads, or creams. Use whatever form you like best, because it's not the form that matters, it's the concentration. Strongest isn't necessarily better. Because it's so drying, you want to find the lowest concentration that helps you. Start with 2.5 percent and go from there. You can buy 10 percent treatments, but they're usually meant for the chest and back, which can tolerate higher concentrations.

Moderate to Severe Acne

There are lots of other options, depending on your level of inflammation, the type of pimples you have (cystic, nodular), and what has or hasn't worked for you in the past. They include prescriptions a dermatologist can give you, such as:

- Topical retinoids (tretinoin, tazarotene, and adapalene), used either alone or mixed with an antibiotic lotion (usually clindamycin or erythromycin).
- Oral antibiotics, such as extended-release minocycline, which only has to be taken once a day (these antibiotics act as anti-inflammatories).
- Oral contraceptives, which often can help—they are what stopped my teenage acne
- Isotretinoin (Accutane), an oral vitamin A derivative that really knocks out severe or stubborn acne. It also is the only medication in the world known to stop the scarring some people experience with acne. Accutane does have more risks associated with it and, because it can cause birth defects, women who use Accutane must register with the drug maker (iPLEDGE is the program), stating that they are not pregnant. Birth-control pills are typically prescribed with Accutane to ensure there are no accidents. Whether you are a candidate for Accutane (and you've tried everything else) is a question for you and your doctor to determine. It can be an incredibly powerful treatment for severe acne, and has changed the lives of many people who could not find solutions in other treatment plans.

Beware: Photodynamic Therapy May Not Be Worth the Pain

If you are impatient and can afford it, there's a procedure called *photodynamic therapy* (PDT) that can jump-start an acne clear-up plan. I'll be honest: It's painful and costly, and probably won't be covered by your health insurance plan.

PDT involves painting your face with a clear liquid acid (ALA or Levulan) that is absorbed by skin cells, especially damaged ones. After a half hour or so, an intense beam of light is used to activate the acid in the cells, which kills the bacteria responsible for the acne. The procedure, which may need to be repeated, can be incredibly painful both during and afterward, and you may experience redness and peeling for a week or two. However, it quickly clears up acne problems, plus, if there are any actinic keratoses, or precancers, around, it wipes them out, too. However, I don't encourage patients to go this route.

Key Dos and Don'ts for Anyone with Acne

This is the basic advice that I find myself repeating over and over, to adults who are dealing with acne for the first time.

- Use a headband to smooth back your hair when you're washing your face, so that you can see and wash every inch.
- Apply spot acne treatments to fresh clean skin, not after you put on your makeup!
- Wait a minute or two for a pimple cream to be absorbed before putting anything else on your face. If it takes any longer, you've used too much.
- Don't mix benzoyl peroxide and moisturizer—you'll dilute the BP to the point of uselessness.
- Wash your makeup brushes; suds them with shampoo, rinse, and hang with the bristles pointing down to air dry.
- If you're using Retin-A or other retinoid treatments, don't bother using them when you need to use benzoyl peroxide. It seems to cancel out retinoids' benefits.

Urban Acne or Urban Myth? Do you really have to worry that your urban life could be giving you acne, too? Air researchers who've looked at mouse skin speculate that ozone and other common air pollutants, like nitric oxide, might make skin more susceptible to allergies and irritation. Of course, it's a huge leap from irritated mouse skin to human acne.

Here's what we do know: If you're a city dweller like me, it makes sense to be extra careful about protecting your skin from UV light, because it reacts with air pollution in ways we're still learning about. On the other hand, if you have acne, don't assume that city air is making your face extra dirty and that you have to superclean it. Overscrubbing is a good way to intensify your acne.

Four Common Breakouts to Break Up

Small white dots or black spots: These little buggers are called *whiteheads* and *blackheads*. Both blackheads and whiteheads are caused by clogged pores; blackheads (open comedones) are open to the air and oxygen oxidizes the sebum and turns it black. *Whiteheads* (closed comedones) are the same lesion closed.

- Break up: A daily face wash with benzoyl peroxide to kill the bacteria is helpful. Use this after your daily cleanser. A good one is Neutrogena Clear Pore Cleanser/Mask. You can also spot treat an area with a salicylic acid formula, like Vichy Normaderm Anti-Blemish Treatment Cream.

Small and red with a white center: Called *pustules*, these start as red dots, but turn into inflamed lesions with a white pus-filled center. Many women get these right before their period when hormone levels are high (yes, they can be hormonally driven). The skin produces too many pimple-causing oils, setting the stage for a clogged pore.

- Break up: If you experience this type of acne, a daily three-step cleansing/toner/moisturizer plan will help keep skin under control. Try Clinique Acne Solutions Clear Skin System Kit. The toner will help exfoliate the skin so that those sticky cells don't clog the pore. A woman can also consider birth-control pills to help regulate hormones and reduce the level of testosterone production, which triggers acne.

Small pink and red bumps: These are called *papules* because they are round, raised bumps. Although they have become inflamed, they don't form whiteheads.

- Break up: Best solution here is to see a dermatologist for a retinoid product, which will unclog pores by removing dead skin cells. It also helps dry up excess oils and reduces acne-causing bacteria. You'd start using a retinoid twice a week and gradually increase to every night.

Large, hard bumps: Big, painful pimples like this are called *nodules* or *cysts,* and they are oil-filled pimples that live deep under the skin, showing up as swollen bumps. These can scar.

- *Break up:* Injections of dilute kenalog, an anti-inflammatory steroid, oral antibiotics, and topical retinoids can come to the rescue here. The injections would go directly into the pimple (this is called an ILK Intra-Lesional kenalog [ILK]). It will dissolve oil and reduce inflammation. Oral antibiotics will help dry deep pimples and prevent new breakouts.

---

acne through the ages

One thing I want to get straight is that for all intents and purposes, acne is acne, whether you're dealing with acne around your period, your pregnancy, your holiday preparations, or your laid-off husband. Sometimes, it helps to get a handle on why acne can surface at particular moments, and how you can best treat it successfully. I will discuss a few acne-generating situations. Bear in mind, however, that the underlying cause of almost all these situations is stress and the reactions that take place in the body as a result, which can be worsened by hormones, genetics, and so on.

Hormonal Acne

If your menstrual periods are a bit quirky (that is, not arriving like clockwork every twenty-eight to thirty-two days), or if you have a disorder called *polycystic ovary syndrome* (PCOS), you may notice what you think is a rash along your chin and jawline. That and extra dark fuzz on your upper lip are hormone-acne giveaways. For some reason, the male hormone, testosterone, is binding more tightly to the androgen receptors in that part of your face, causing the bumps; you'll need to see a doctor for blood tests to check your hormone levels.

Even if those levels are normal, birth control pills, which have the advantage of reducing circulating testosterone levels, can help clear up your face. A good new one: Yaz, which is FDA-approved to treat acne, thanks to an active ingredient that blocks androgen. If the bumps are inflamed and deep, or cystic, they may be more stubborn. In that case, you might need a retinoid and either an antibiotic or an antiandrogen. You'll also need to address the extra hair. Don't shave! Women's facial skin is too delicate; you can create more inflammatory lesions. More important, I think shaving one's face is deeply emotional; it's defeminizing, and puts a hole in your entire sense of self as a woman. Plucking is no better because it produces red bumps. Your best bets are electrolysis or laser hair removal.

Product Acne

Many cosmetics are designed to be noncomedogenic, meaning they won't clog your pores. I rarely see product acne (it's much less common than you might think) and, in fact, when someone believes she is reacting to a particular product, in all likelihood it's something else. The psychological attachment to the product being to blame, however, means by stopping using it, she is less stressed out about it. It's possible that your skin may react to an unsuspected ingredient. To pinpoint the product, keep a skin diary, noting down anything new in your regimen—soaps, cleansers, serums, treatments, makeup, *everything*. Stop using one of them for five to seven days and see if your skin improves; if not, move on to the next. One product that is often problematic and not an automatic *aha!* is sunscreen. Patients sometimes tell me they are really stressed because they've got these little bumps or blackheads on their forehead. Turns out they used a sunscreen one or two days earlier that wasn't oil free. Make sure you've got an oil-free face formula with a good UV protector like zinc oxide or titanium dioxide.

Since product acne may take three to six weeks to clear completely, try an over-the-counter salicylic acid peel to help calm any inflammation. Or get a prescription for a topical mix of benzoyl peroxide and clindamycin and use it all over your face.

Q: What do you think of three-step acne treatment kits like ProActiv Solution?

A: What many people like about these three-step kits is that the products are all put together for you, and that it can be cheaper than buying them individually. Typically, you get either a cleanser-toner-moisturizer or a cleanser-toner-treatment, and one or two of the products will have benzoyl peroxide or salicylic acid in them, which really help acne. The drawback is that often one of the three treatments won't suit you, so that can be a waste of money.

I actually think ProActiv is good for mild acne, though it's expensive. Again, if it doesn't work, don't keep trying more and more stuff. At that point, you need derm-strength.

Big-Event Acne

Weddings and speeches can send stress soaring like nothing else. From your mother's suggestions for everything from the place settings to the flowers to the realization that you're about to marry a grown man who still plays video games, weddings can offer a host of stresses. The same goes for big presentations for work. The last thing you need is waking to fresh pimples on your face, but it probably will happen at some point. Even happy occasions can be stress-tests that result in skin emergencies. If you have a morning-before disaster on your face, a dermatologist can fix it with an injection of anti-inflammatory steroid. This is a one-time emergency spot treatment; it's not for regular use. If you've got a big event coming up and know from past experience you'll probably have a pimple coming up right then, too, get a prescription for Vanoxide HC (2 percent benzoyl peroxide with 0.5 hydrocortisone cream), so you're not caught unprepared.

Pregnancy Acne

If you're lucky enough not to have had pimples in the past, any that you get now probably won't be severe. For the acne-prone, being pregnant can be a challenge: If your current treatments are a threat to your unborn baby, you'll have to discontinue them and, as a result, your acne may get worse. Don't give up! You can use pregnancy-safe acne remedies: prescription topical erythromycin or azeleic acid, or over-the-counter topical salicylic acid. Though they haven't been specifically tested during pregnancy, they're FDA-approved and their relative risk is quite low. Be sure to discuss it with your obstetrician, as well as your skin doctor.

Over-Forty Acne

By the time you get into your forties, you want acne to be a thing of the past so you can focus on fighting wrinkles. Alas, women in their forties break out, too. Maybe you've started taking a new medicine like lithium for depression or an iodine drug for an underactive thyroid. These and some other meds, including corticosteroids, epilepsy medications, and antituberculosis drugs, can lead to skin eruptions. Tell your doctors about your reaction, so that together you can figure out a treatment plan that doesn't interfere with your primary problem.

Q: What are heat treatments like Zeno good for?

A: The directions for Zeno primarily recommend it for pimples that are just beginning to appear—it's a nip-them-in-the-bud approach—but not for anything really red, hard, and angry, such as severe nodular or cystic acne. The company also doesn't recommend it for blackheads and whiteheads. Frankly, I don't recommend Zeno at all. Use benzoyl peroxide. It does the same thing Zeno claims to do—kill off *P. acnes* bacteria—and it's far cheaper.

Dermatologists sometimes use lasers to treat acne, which does work well, but the treatment must be repeated and are painful. Another option is a new machine called *Isolaz,* which isn't laser therapy. It's a vacuum that sucks out gunk from the pimples, then emits a strong blue (painless) light that helps destroy the acne-causing bacteria, sloughing the oils and dead skin cells away. This light may also shrink the sebaceous gland, so that oil production is reduced. Isolaz can also be used to treat uneven skin tone, sun-damaged skin, facial redness, veins, and unwanted hair. You can't do this at home; seek a dermatologist who is using this form of laser therapy.

If pimples have joined your wrinkles, now may be a good time to start on a topical retinoid like *tazarotene* (Tazarac). Start with a low concentration, and use cream rather than gel. The plus: It can help eradicate fine lines.

And remember that being over forty doesn't exclude you from maintaining a daily skin regimen. Check your products, both cleansing and makeup, to be sure they are noncomedogenic. Wash your face twice a day as prescribed earlier in the book: If you want to add benzoyl peroxide or salicylic acid to your routine, start with one (benzoyl peroxide or salicylic acid) and use it for two to three weeks. If that doesn't do the trick, add the other (for example, do a benzoyl peroxide wash and salicylic toner or spot treatment). Don't forget to moisturize! All too often I see patients who have overtreated and overdried out their skin to the point at which they start the inflammatory cycle all over again. Be good to your skin. Nourish it. Hydrate it. Keep it clean and supple.

Q: What concealers and foundations do you recommend to camouflage a pimple?

A: The simplest answer is not bargain brands. It's worth going to a department store or shopping online and spending a little more for these because it's tricky to make a noncomedogenic foundation that camouflages well without being opaque and thick. The same goes for concealers. Cheap ones tend to be gloppy. Just double-check that they're noncomedogenic. I particularly like these.

Clinique

Perfectly Real Makeup (liquid or compact)

RepairWear Anti-Aging SPF 15 foundation

Laura Mercier www.LauraMercier.com

Secret Camouflage concealer

Oil-Free Foundation

Mac Cosmetics www.maccosmetics.com

Studio Finish SPF35 concealer

Select Moisture Blend SPF15 foundation

Studio Tech foundation

Shiseido

The Makeup Dual Balancing foundation SPF 17

Before we move on to the topic of skin cancer in the next chapter, let me cover a few other common skin conditions that I see every day in my office. Most of these are best left to dermatological treatments, and an in-depth discussion of these is beyond the scope of this book. Use the following summary as a starting point if you suffer from any of these conditions. You will then feel better informed when you consult with your dermatologist.

Eczema

Also called *atopic dermatis,* this chronic skin disorder, which tends to run in families, involves scaly and itchy rashes, and is often due to a sensitivity in the skin much like an allergy. This allergy leads to short-term and long-term inflammation (yes, the same inflammatory response we've been covering since the beginning of the book). Eczema is very common in infants and young children, and in adults can be chronic. People with eczema often aggravate the condition by continuing to scratch the affected area, which causes it to thicken and thicker skin is itchier. Treating eczema starts with halting the itch-scratch cycle and usually includes a dry-skin care routine. This would entail using very mild cleansers, avoiding washcloths, and being diligent about applying rich moisturizers to the skin while it's still damp right out of the shower. Topical anti-inflammatories such as cortisone creams can also help. Several treatment options are available depending on how bad your particular eczema is, and by your figuring out if there is a specific irritant triggering the condition. Your doctor can help you with this.

Free Skin Tip

If your skin's barrier function is healthy, your risk for skin conditions rooted in out-of-control inflammation is lower. Ease up on your skin; be gentle to it and use sensitive-skin formulas when you wash, moisturize, and apply makeup. And don't forget about switching to laundry detergents that are fragrance-free and dye-free. Choose fragrance-free fabric softener and cut back on colognes and perfumes.

Psoriasis

Various forms of psoriasis exist but, in general, psoriasis is a chronic skin disorder characterized by periodic flare-ups of sharply defined red plaques, covered by a silvery, flaky surface. In the most common form, called *plaque psoriasis,* thick red patches appear most often on the elbows, knees, scalp, lower back, buttocks, and belly button. Other areas can also be affected, including nails and body folds.

We don't know exactly what causes psoriasis, but it appears that a combination of factors contribute to its development. Basically, psoriasis starts with inflammation in the skin that prompts new skin cells to develop. The process starts in the *basal* (bottom) layer of the *epidermis,* where keratinocytes are made. *Keratinocytes* are epidermal skin cells that produce *keratin,* a tough protein that helps form hair, nails, and skin. In normal cell growth, keratinocytes grow and move from the bottom layer to the skin's surface and shed unnoticed. This process takes about a month.

In people with psoriasis, the keratinocytes multiply very rapidly and travel from the basal layer to the surface in about three to four days. The skin cannot shed these cells quickly enough, so they build up, leading to thick, dry plaques. Silvery, flaky areas of dead skin build up on the surface of the plaques. The underlying skin layer *(dermis),* which contains the nerves, blood, and lymphatic vessels, becomes red and swollen.

There has been a great deal of research on psoriasis and stress, and there are currently a variety of treatments available, including oral prescriptive medication. The stress can also be local, such as the stress caused by trauma to the skin. This could be as simple as the pressure from sitting on your butt all day, getting a cut or burn, or leaning on your elbows. As with any itchy, scaly skin, the more you scratch, the itchier it gets. This, then, causes the epidermis to get thicker and as a result, itchier. Breaking the cycle of scratching the area is key, as is controlling inflammation and any underlying cause of inflammation.

Scratch! Scratch! Scratch!

The more you scratch your skin, the itchier it gets. The epidermis will get thicker, and as a result, *itchier*. Break the cycle. If you can't help but scratch, pick, and play with an inflamed or scabbed area, try an over-the-counter hydrocortisone cream twice a day. You can also try ice, covering the area with a band aid, or look for an over-the-counter antiitch product that contains pramoxine, such as Sarna Sensitive.

Q: Are spider veins hereditary and impossible to treat?

A: Sorry, but you can't blame your parents for these veins, which can be red, blue, or purple. Pregnancy, birth control pills, and trauma to the leg, such as surgery or a car accident, can cause them. (No, you can't get them from crossing your legs too often.) Unfortunately, some manufacturers of spider-vein therapies claim vitamin K is the secret weapon, as it can constrict blood vessels to make them less visible, but its molecules are simply too big to get through your skin's layers. Even if it did reach the veins it wouldn't do anything: Vitamin K is involved in the clotting cascade when you are actively bleeding. The best way to tackle spider veins is with *sclerotherapy.* A doctor will inject tiny amounts of a solution (hypertonic saline or sotradechol are among the most popular) that causes the veins to swell shut. About 95 percent of patients see an improvement after one to three sclerotherapy treatments.

Rosacea

The hallmarks of this skin condition, which affects adults after the age of about thirty, is redness on the forehead, nose, cheeks, and chin. Fair-skinned people who blush or become flushed easily may be more at risk for rosacea. Some people develop a ruddy appearance and blood vessels can become visible, as well as pimples in the red area. It can also affect the eyes, making them irritated and watery. Lots of people who think they have rosacea, however, simply have sun damage. Only about one in ten patients I see who think they have rosacea actually has it. In the general population, about 14 million Americans have rosacea.

Several theories exist to explain the still-unknown cause of rosacea, but one truth is certain: Inflammation is at the heart of the problem. What we don't know is what triggers that inflammation. It could be a generalized disorder of the blood vessels, or something more specific such as microscopic skin mites, psychological stress, sun exposure, weather, alcohol, hormones, spicy foods, heavy exercise, hot tubs, fragrances, allergies, and so on. It may also be a combination of factors. Symptoms as well as triggers can vary considerably from person to person, and knowing what activates your rosacea is step one in preventing and controlling it. There is no cure yet for rosacea, but there are treatments available such as topical retinoids, creams, and oral antibiotics aimed at decreasing redness, inflammation, and acne bumps.

Your dermatologist can help you choose the best treatment plan for you given the characteristics of your individual rosacea. If you suspect you could have this condition, don't try to take care of it on your own. There is not much by way of over-the-counter remedies that really work and, if left untreated, it can progress to the point that large blood vessels and pus-filled pimples appear. Clearly, this is inflammation maxed out! To make matters worse, the disorder also can cause the nose to become bulbous and swollen as the tissue thickens, a condition called *rhinophyma*. This explains the famous nose and appearance of W. C. Fields in his later years.

Cold Sores

Cold sores are caused by the herpes virus, which has been in human bloodlines for millennia. It remains dormant in bodies infected with this virus until it's activated by any number of things, including stress, an illness, fever, sun exposure, sleep deprivation, and so on. In fact, anything that stresses the body—whether physical, emotional, or psychological—can set off a cold sore's development as the immune system takes a dive. And, as with rosacea, knowing your personal triggers is key to preventing and controlling the virus's actions. Usually, people feel a tingling sensation at first, and that's when it's important to have a remedy on hand to help control its severity. Antiviral prescription oral medication and topical creams are available; your individual protocol will depend on how frequently you get cold sores. The creams don't work nearly as well as the antiviral meds. If you have more than five episodes a year, you can take suppressive therapy every day.

Q: My jewelry seems to irritate me. I get a little red rash every time I wear certain pieces. What's going on?

A: Contact allergies are common, especially from accessories, including watches, costume jewelry, silver, and gold. The culprit is nickel in the jewelry, even in so-called silver and gold bling that is not 100 percent pure or solid. The solution is to stick with platinum and stainless steel. You can spot treat any rash with an over-the-counter hydrocortisone cream once per day until it disappears. You can also try painting clear nail polish on the back of any questionable jewelry; this will create a thin defensive barrier. If metal parts on your jeans are giving you trouble on your belly, cover the metal parts with moleskin or duct tape. This can actually survive a few trips to the laundry.

Q: I've had little tiny bumps, some of them red, on the backs of my upper arms and on my butt for years. They don't hurt or itch, but I don't like them. What are they and can I get rid of them?

A: It's been estimated that up to 50 percent of the global adult population—and 50 to 80 percent of adolescents—has this harmless skin condition called *keratosis pilaris*. It's especially visible those who are fair-skinned, and it's commonly found on the upper arms, buttocks, and thighs. The cause? Small, thick keratin plugs in the hair follicles. Gently removing the plugs without irritating the skin is key, and can be tricky. If you get it in adolescence, it may go away by adulthood. Prescription-strength lactic acid, glycolic acid, and 10 to 40 percent urea in a cream or spray are all helpful. On your own, you can try using an over-the-counter, glycolic acid-based exfoliant, and moisturize, which also helps.

Q: Is there anything that can be done for red, purplish spots? I have one right on the side of my face that's about the size of a dime, and I've tried to cover it up with makeup but I'd rather see it gone entirely.

A: More than likely, what you see is a grouping of tiny blood vessels or broken capillaries (called a *spider angioma*). This grouping can be caused by trauma, genetics, sun exposure, or you may have been born with it. Luckily, a dermatologist can laser it away for you and it won't come back. You may need to repeat the laser session two or three times, about one month apart, but it's quick, noninvasive, and pretty painless.

9

skin cancer basics

What You Need to Know about Sunscreen and Cancer Prevention

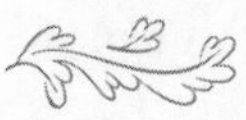

A book about skin beauty cannot avoid this topic, especially today when more and more *young* people seek treatment for precancerous lesions and surfacing cancerous cells. Nothing ages your skin like cancer. The physical toll cancer takes on your skin as well as the emotional toll it takes on your beauty confidence is far bigger than anyone realizes, until it happens to her.

One would think the main issue with skin cancer is worrying about how serious it is, and whether or not it's the type that can spread to other parts of the body. In reality, most women fret about how the skin will look after the cancer has been removed. They assume it can be treated, especially when detected early, and they don't want to be left with an ugly scar. Just being diagnosed with skin cancer makes them feel old. I have a sixty-seven-year-old patient who has seven basal and squamous cell carcinomas (I'll explain what these are later in this chapter) and multiple excisions. He says he feels like he's falling apart—that his *skin* is falling apart and the rest will soon follow.

Feeling one's own mortality like this is not a confidence booster. No one can ignore the fact that we all get older, but we try to avoid acknowledging this reality until suddenly a diagnosis like skin cancer emerges. It's remarkable, however, to think that your skin has been dealing with UV-induced sun dam-

Putting into Perspective

Skin cancer is the most common of all cancers, accounting for nearly half of all cancers in the United States. An estimated 40 to 50 percent of Americans who live to age sixty-five will have skin cancer at least once—the most common type being a basal cell carcinoma, which accounts for more than 90 percent of all skin cancers. Most of the more than 1 million cases of nonmelanoma skin cancer diagnosed yearly in the United States are considered to be sun-related. In 2007, *melanoma*, the most serious type of skin cancer, accounted for about 59,940 cases of skin cancer. And of the 10,850 people who die of skin cancer each year, most (about 8,110) are caused by melanoma.

age for years and, at a certain age, your repair mechanisms simply don't work as well. That age, by the way, is different in everyone, and no one can tell you when or even if you will get skin cancer.

It helps to bear in mind that getting skin cancer is not a sign of falling apart or even oldness. Realize that skin is often the first to take a hit because it's been taking hits for a very long time out there on the front lines. Sixty-seven is not old, and neither is seventy, seventy-five, or even eighty. Old is a measure of how you *feel*—period. No matter your age, you can still be youthful. After all, the point of this book is to look as young as you feel, right?

With this in mind, let's explore skin cancer basics and the rundown on sunscreens. I'll start by explaining why we take to the sun so much, and may have a hard time protecting ourselves from its long-term ruins.

if sun's so bad for you, why does it feel soooo good?

Unless you've spent the last two decades exploring the Antarctic, you know the sun's ultraviolet light is pretty much skin's mortal enemy. So, why *does* it feel so good? That's not an idle question: UV light may wind up joining the ranks of alcohol, cigarettes, cocaine, and other drugs as an addictive substance. In fact, when researchers questioned avid beach-goers about it, their answers indicated signs of substance abuse. The sun-lovers, or perhaps, tanaholics, said they thought about tanning first thing in the morning, felt they should cut back, were guilty about their habit, and got annoyed if anyone criticized it. Deeply understanding the risks made no difference; even if a family member had had skin cancer, they were likely to keep right on tanning.

While it's true that the skin produces endorphins, notably beta-endorphins, in response to broad-spectrum (natural) light, the feel-good sensation that accompanies being in the sun is likely a psychological response. Think about it: Most people associate sunbathing with vacations, time away from school or work, tropical islands, honeymoons . . . a relaxed state of mind. In fact, when tanaholics are asked why they seek out the sun, many say "to relax." In animals, stress boosts the desire for addictive drugs; in humans, it inhibits the part of the brain that normally puts the brakes on risky behavior. Looking at it from an evolutionary perspective also helps make sense of this; for millennia we roamed about the land and spent a great deal more time outside than inside.

> ***Do You Break for the Sun?***
>
> If so, you could be a *heliomaniac*—someone addicted to the sun. *Helio* means sun, and *maniac*, well . . .

Today, most people live more confined lives, staying and working indoors for much of the day. Some of us rarely see the sun anymore thanks to long working hours that have us commuting before dawn and home after dark. What happens is that your psychological reaction to being in the great outdoors and sun triggers your body to release feel-good hormones from the inside. Meanwhile, the endorphins created locally in your skin act as anti-inflammatories. They also may help boost your natural collagen and protect against wrinkles, acne, and UV-derived sun damage.

The research aiming to understand the addiction factor of tanning and seeking the warmth of the sun is still in its infancy, but one cannot deny the feel-good sensations that accompany many people's reaction to sunlight. Numerous studies have demonstrated how sunlight can lessen the symptoms of seasonal affected disorder (SAD; see page 220) and depression. Much of sunlight's effect on mood is related to the visible light that hits your *eyes*. Remember, cycles of light and dark affect the production of certain hormones like melatonin, which in turn says a lot about our biological rhythms and moods.

Q: What's the difference between a mole and a wart? Can they become cancerous and are they easy to remove?

A: Moles and warts are two entirely different things. Moles are growths on the skin composed of *melanocytes*—cells in the epidermis that produce the pigment melanin and give skin its natural color—whereas warts are caused by the *human papilloma virus* (HPV). For this reason, warts are contagious and can be spread through direct contact with HPV; there are more than 60 kinds of HPV, some of which lead to warts on the skin. The types that cause these benign skin warts do not cause cancer. HPV stimulates quick growth of cells on the skin's outer layer. In most cases, common warts appear on the fingers, hands, feet, and toes (but they really can crop up anywhere). Certain types of HPV also can cause warts to appear in the genital area or cause genital cancers, particularly cervical cancer. Different subtypes of HPV, however, cause genital warts than cause cervical cancer. Genital HPV is the most common sexually transmitted disease in the United States.

There are plenty of treatments for benign skin warts, and over-the-counter wart removal kits work well for most people. For a troubling wart, a dermatologist can prescribe a cream like Aldara, remove it through freezing (cryotherapy), minor surgery, or apply of a chemical substance that literally kills off the wart.

You won't find over-the-counter kits for removing moles, on the other hand. These usually require minor surgery, and you could be trading a mole for a scar. Very few moles become cancer, but because moles often result from sun exposure (the sun triggers the melanocytes to produce more pigment), it's important to keep an eye on them and get any checked out that look different from the others. About one out of every ten people has at least one unusual mole that looks different from an ordinary mole. The medical term for these atypical moles is *dysplastic nevi,* and while they are not cancer themselves, they can become cancer. People with these types of moles are more likely to develop melanoma. Approximately 20 percent of melanomas start in a mole (but this doesn't mean that 20 percent of moles turn into melanomas).

Remember, moles can be beauty marks. Don't ever try to take off a mole or, for that matter, a birthmark yourself! See a doctor before doing any self-surgery in the bathroom.

If you just can't stop tanning, start keeping a journal of your feelings, and try to pinpoint the reasons for your habit. If stress jumps out, try exchanging your UV fix for a walk in a natural setting or a try lightbox therapy. You can purchase or rent a light box that emits visible light (with UV filters that block the radiation). Bright-light therapy has many uses, such as aiding in jet lag, seasonal blues, low mood, fatigue, and resetting your circadian rhythm (*see* SAD box for more).

Are You SAD? Look into the Light!

If you live in an area characterized by lots of overcast days in the winter months, you may have been a victim of seasonal affective disorder, or SAD, a mood disorder associated with episodes of depression and related to seasonal variations of light.

Symptoms of SAD include exhaustion and chronic sleepiness, the need to sleep nine or more hours a night, feelings of sadness and depression, excessive eating and weight gain, and powerful carbohydrate cravings, especially for sugary and/or starchy foods. You might also have a difficult time concentrating. Often these symptoms emerge during the fall and winter months as the days grow shorter, darker, and light becomes an infrequent visitor. They then disappear as spring turns over a new leaf, and longer, brighter days herald the onset of summer, which invigorates people's zest for life and squelches any signs of depression.

Because our internal clocks, rhythms, and regulators are heavily influenced by exposure to light, it's no surprise that one of the main causes of SAD is prolonged deprivation of adequate sunlight that our bodies need to stay on track. The hormones that affect mood, energy, and even food cravings can become imbalanced. Hence, the ways to prevent and/or treat SAD include arranging for exposure to light every day (natural sunlight, or using lightbox therapy), staying active and maintaining routine physical exercise, and scheduling a midwinter vacation in a warm, sunny place.

Ever been curious about exactly why those feel-good rays are so bad for your skin? Here's how photoaging, or aging caused by the sun, accumulates:

A is for aging, B is for burning. There are two key types of ultraviolet radiation—UVA and UVB light—and both ravage skin, damaging its DNA, provoking cancer, and accelerating wrinkles, sagging, and other signs of time. UVA has been dubbed the *aging ray* because, over time, the dermis damage it does produces wrinkles and pigment changes. UVB, the *burning ray*, triggers inflammation and dilates blood vessels—sunburn. Any time you get tanned, it means you've damaged your skin. Your body has upped its production of melanin pigment, which acts as a UV filter, in an attempt to shield skin from photodamage.

Skin fights back. As sunlight penetrates your skin, it batters your DNA. UVB attacks DNA directly, UVA also damages and cells and DNA but penetrates even more deeply, which is why it's dubbed the silent wrinkler, as it goes much deeper than the other rays to cause a delayed tan, delayed wrinkling, and delayed skin cancer. These rays injure a host of cells, including *fibroblasts,* which produce collagen and elastin. The skin's stress response system signals an alert and defensive cells rush in to undo the harm, but the result is never quite like new. What's more, both types of UV appear to eventually suppress the immune system, which may be a factor in melanoma, the most serious kind of skin cancer.

Sag sets in and spots surface. Gradually, collagen breaks down and becomes disorganized and abnormal elastin increases, so skin loses its stretchiness and becomes looser, saggy, less resilient, and more wrinkled. Production of *melanocytes,* skin's pigment-producing cells, becomes erratic, making skin tone uneven, blotchy, and spotted.

Red spreads. UV rays encourage the creation of new blood vessels, which may give you a sprinkling of *telangiectasias*—spidery red spots—and help skin cancers form. Skin usually thins with age, but regularly sun-exposed skin on the back of your neck will get thick and leathery as a defensive reaction to UV light.

My Four-Step Wrinkle-Stopping Strategy

Granted, it's tough to battle an invisible foe like the sun for years. But wouldn't you like to be the one among your friends who always looks the youngest and has the best skin? Here's my system.

- **Always seek shade.** It reduces UV by 50 to 95 percent. Sit under a tree or beach umbrella, walk on the shady side of the street, and park yourself on the protected side of a train, bus, or car for midday rides (glass doesn't block UVA). You may also want to check out UV-protection shields for cars (3M Company makes them) if you are a frequent commuter during daylight hours. Avoidance is your number-one tactic, especially between ten in the morning and four in the afternoon, and near reflective surfaces (sand, water, snow). Even when it's overcast, 80 percent of UV light zips right through clouds.
- **Cover your body.** I know what you're thinking: Who in their right mind wears a lot of clothes at the pool? Or on a hike? Be creative. At the seashore, when you're not in the water, wrap a sarong or beach towel around your lower half, pull on a T-shirt, plop on a wide-brimmed hat, and wear your sunglasses (they're nonnegotiable; you can burn your corneas, and who wants crow's feet?). For sports, invest in a few pieces of lightweight clothing specially made with an ultraviolet protection factor, or UPF. A UPF of 50 means only one-fiftieth of the sun's UV rays pass through it. Or use a laundry product with TinosorbFD to increase the UPF of your clothes; it'll last through repeated washings. (Go to www.RealAge.com for sources.)
- **Think one teaspoon, two shot glasses.** Sunscreen only works if you use enough of it. Before you head outdoors, smooth one teaspoon's worth of broad-spectrum sunscreen with SPF 30 or higher on your face and apply at least three ounces—two shot glasses full—of sunscreen to your body.

On beach days, I usually slather on sunscreen when I'm naked to make sure I'm totally covered before I slip into a bathing suit. And don't forget your ears, neck, backs of hands, feet, and lips (use at least an SPF 30 lip balm). P.S. There is no such thing as a base tan that protects you from further sun damage. A base tan can prevent burning because it's your skin's defense mechanism against burning, but you'll still suffer damage.

- **Set your cell phone alarm.** Set it to ring two to three hours later, and reapply sunscreen when it goes off. Whenever you come out of the pool or off the volleyball court, reapply even if you put on sweatproof or water-resistant sunscreen.

My Favorite Sunscreen

For my face, I personally prefer Anthelios XL 50 Fluide Extreme (made by La Roche-Posay). There are seventeen FDA-approved sunscreen ingredients. Most are chemicals that absorb UV radiation; they take about thirty minutes to take effect, and some can irritate sensitive skin. However, two—zinc oxide and titanium dioxide—are physical blockers that block UVA and UVB. They go to work instantly, and won't irritate skin (this makes them ideal for kids). When I run out of my Anthelios, any sunscreen with zinc or titanium will do, but at the right percentage. I look for a broad-spectrum sunscreen that contains at least 9 percent zinc or titanium, such as Neutrogena Sensitive Skin Sunscreen. Micronized zinc oxide appears to be a better UVA filter than micronized titanium dioxide so, given a choice, opt for zinc.

For the best protection, you need a broad-spectrum sunscreen that works for both UVA and UVB rays. The problem is, a recent study found that 18 percent of U.S. sunscreens fell short in providing UVA protection, even though they were labeled broad-spectrum. For UVB coverage, just choose a product with SPF 30 or higher, which filters out 97 percent of UVB. Getting UVA coverage is trickier, because the FDA just recently set standards for informing consumers on UVA protection. Manufacturers won't be forced to upgrade their labeling until around May 2009. By then, they will have to indicate on the label the strength of their products' UVA protection level by using a four-star rating system. The SPF number on the label will relate to the UVB and the four-star rating will relate to the UVA. The new regulations also change the highest SPF values from 30+ to 50+. So go for a four-star formula (and at least 30+).

Six Sunscreen Tips That You Don't Know

- If you're dark-skinned, choose chemical sunscreens over zinc and titanium formulas, as the mineral-based ones may give you a whitish hue.
- If a sunscreen makes your skin sting, itch, or break out, the likely culprits are PABA, benzophenone-3, or octyl methoxycinnamate; switch to a formula without those ingredients. If you are sensitive to any of these chemicals, switch to any of the zinc oxide or titanium dioxide varieties.
- Apply indoors, about thirty minutes before you go out in the sun.
- Ignore promises of "all-day protection" and "water-resistant"; they are not reliable. Reapply all sunscreens at least every two to three hours and right after you've been sweating a lot or swimming.
- There's an expiration date on sunscreens. Check it and toss old ones (most last up to two years).
- Don't store sunscreens in the glove compartment of your car—heat degrades them.

Don't forget to protect your lips, hands, and the tops of those ears. These are common areas for skin cancer that people forget about. Speaking of hands, nothing shows your age more than your hands, probably because we expose them to the elements every day and forget to treat them with some TLC! One of my favorite antiaging hand creams on the market is right at your local drugstore: Cetaphil Therapeutic Hand Cream with Shea Butter. It feels wonderful on your skin, soaks in quickly, and is very accessible.

Why a *Little* Sun Can Be a Good Thing

Don't be phobic of the sun. All this talk about skin cancer and using sunscreen every day is not meant to instill so much fear in you that you avoid sunlight at all costs. Even though my kids go off to summer camp with bottles of sunscreen they know to use diligently, by the end of summer they have some tan lines. But I know that they didn't burn. And that's key.

We need the sun to some degree in our lives; in fact, it's a vital part of our health and longevity. For some people, especially those in northern climates where regular sunlight is less frequent, the health benefits from the sun might outweigh the risk of skin cancer. Exposure to natural sunlight is a surefire way to lift a blue mood, perhaps by boosting brain levels of *serotonin*. Sunlight reduces the need for postoperative painkillers, as patients in sunny rooms feel less stress and pain after surgery. And the sun can help improve certain skin conditions, such as psoriasis.

Burning It Up

Between 1999 and 2004, the number of Americans who got sunburned *increased* from 31.8 percent to 33.7 percent. Among Caucasian women, whose fair skin makes them extravulnerable to turning lobster red, the numbers rose even higher: from 35.3 to 39.6 percent. This trend needs reversing.

The debate about vitamin D deficiency in the general population is growing. A number of studies have found that higher vitamin D, which the body makes using sunlight, protects against some cancers and illnesses, such as rickets, bone-thinning osteoporosis, and diabetes. It also helps the body's immune system work properly. Certain foods and vitamin supplements contain vitamin D, but the main source for the body is the sun. It only takes ten to twenty minutes of sunlight a few times a week to make plenty of vitamin D. Still, if you spend most of your time indoors and/or live in the northern half of the country, producing enough D can be problematic, especially in winter.

The best way to compromise between these two competing effects (good versus bad health benefits) is to maintain a voice of reason. I don't expect my patients to coat themselves in sunblock every single day from head to toe. I also don't expect people to shy away from the sun, lock themselves inside, close the window shades, and turn into vampires. What kind of living would that be? Just be smart about the sun and your skin. A little bit of common sense goes a long way.

There Is a Perfect Tan Love the skin you were born in. I've learned to love being pale, even though when I was a teenager playing playing beach volleyball, being tan was part of my life, and I didn't know any better. I've been making up for it ever since. Still, lots of people simply prefer how they look with a tan. Fine! Just make sure it's perfect. And the *only* way to get a perfect tan—no strap marks, no red zones, just even, glowing gold—is with a sunless tanner. Whether it's professionally sprayed on or DIY at home, they work amazingly well. The active ingredient in most of the do-it-yourselfers is a simple nontoxic sugar called *dihydroxyacetone* (DHA). Just remember that these surface tans afford no UV protection, so you still need to slather on your favorite sunscreen.

skin cancer's toll—and how to stop it

Most Americans don't take skin cancer that seriously, probably because the vast majority of cases are both treatable and curable.

However, we forget the physical scars skin cancer leaves and the emotional toll it takes on a woman's beauty confidence. Take Kate, a lively, pretty fifty-year-old who recently became a patient. She had a spot on her nose that another physician had lasered a couple of times, but the spot kept coming back. She came to me for a second opinion and I did a biopsy—removed some cells and sent them to a lab. The spot turned out to be melanoma, the most dangerous kind of skin cancer. Taking it out was an ordeal for Kate: A plastic surgeon had to use skin from her forehead to patch up the hole (noses don't have much extra skin). For weeks, Kate wore sunglasses and a hat pulled low over her face. She said she felt vulnerable, ugly, and disfigured (even though she wasn't). And for the first time, she said, she felt old.

That's a frequent reaction to skin cancer, even to basal-cell and squamous-cell cancers, which usually aren't life threatening, but removing them can sometimes leave sizable scars. Getting skin cancer is synonymous with growing old in many people's minds and can deliver a big hit to one's self-esteem. Patients will say, "My skin was my best feature. What do I do now that the whole world can see I've had cancer?" Feelings of bewilderment, sadness that your body let you down, worries over scarring, fear of future cancers—or, with melanoma, of dying—are very common.

Skin Cancer Doesn't Discriminate

The melanin pigment in dark skin acts like a weak sunscreen, although it blocks more UVB than UVA. This doesn't mean that people with dark skin, such as African Americans and Native Americans, are immune to skin cancer. They're not, and their skin's inherent screen isn't nearly strong enough to keep them safe. This mistaken belief helps explain why skin cancer is often diagnosed so late in dark-skinned people, making it much harder to cure.

Treat Your Cancer—and Your Psyche

If you've just been diagnosed with skin cancer, what you need most besides a lot of good doctoring is a little sympathy. Then be proactive. It's the best way to counter the hit to your self-confidence and to prevent a cancer from aging you. The silver lining in dealing with skin cancer is you will begin to take better care of your skin and yourself. When I treat patients in their twenties, thirties, and forties with basal-cell carcinomas, it can be a blessing in disguise—a wake-up call for them to start protecting themselves from the sun. Here's a brief summary of what you can expect; your doctor can give you more specific details related to your type of skin cancer.

If you have a basal cell or squamous cell skin cancer, there are several ways to remove it:

- Scraping and burning (known as *curettage* and *electrodesiccation*), which involves scraping away the tumor, and then burning any remaining cancer cells. This is used for superficial basal cell and squamous cell carcinoma *in situ*—cancers that have not progressed or moved out of the area in question. The doctor will also remove a bit of healthy tissue to prevent a recurrence.
- Freezing away the tumor with liquid nitrogen (*cryosurgery*).
- And surgery, which I believe is usually the best option. It means a lab can test the tissue to make sure every bit of cancer was removed, ensuring you have *clean margins*, and has the best five-year cure rate: 95 percent or better for basal cells.

If surgery is the choice for your type of cancer, assuming the cancer isn't too big, your doctor will probably remove it in the office, using a local anesthesia. Even when a spot looks small on the surface, it may be wide and/or deep underneath, so it's not always possible to tell how large the excision will be in advance. Your doctor will choose the best option based on your particular type of cancer. With surgery, you'll have stitches for a week or two, and a scar will develop. Four to six weeks later, your doctor should check to make sure your body isn't pumping out too much collagen at the scar site, which can produce a *hypertrophic* scar, one that is raised about half an inch and is often itchy and uncomfortable.

To help minimize scarring and ensure full cancer removal, one technique used on the face and ears for both basal and squamous cell carcinomas is called Mohs micrographic surgery. This removes the cancer layer by layer, checking at each stage to see if the margins are clear, and saving as much tissue as possible. It requires special training and the presence of a lab pathologist to check the removed tissue for cancer cells, but it can be done in a doctor's office under local anesthesia. Five-year cure rates are 99 percent.

Time really does heal, and both your skin and your self-esteem will regroup.

Q: My mom is in her early sixties and she's had chronic skin problems, both basal cell and squamous cell spots removed routinely. She has spent much of her life in the sun, so I know it's a result of her addiction to tanning, plus the fact she's got fair skin like me. Am I doomed as her daughter to have the same problems?

A: You are not "doomed," so don't panic. *Your* lifestyle choices, not your mother's, will factor more into your risk for getting skin cancer than your genetics. Take note now and learn from your mom's experience, especially since you have the same skin tone and sensitivity to the sun.

Five Ways to Shrink Scars

- **Massage.** Believe it or not, if you gently massage the healing area a couples of times per day about a month after the stitches are out, it helps remodel collagen, breaking it up newly forming collagen and helping reduce scarring. Don't bother massaging gel caps of vitamin E into a scar to make it fade; it won't. Scar therapies that I have found to be pretty helpful are Curad Scar Therapy and Scarguard. Any silicone sheet will work decently.
- **Pressure.** You can buy and apply pressure bandages with sheets of silicone gel that help keep a scar from growing too big.
- **Lasers.** Bumpy scars can sometimes be smoothed out with a laser. Size counts—the smaller, the better.
- **Steroids.** Scars that heal badly, becoming large and lumpy, can be treated with a laser to reduce their redness, then injected monthly with a steroid for two to six months.
- **Do-overs.** Misshapen scars can sometimes be improved with a do-over if they're not too big and not in a busy location. Back scars, for instance, generally aren't good candidates because they tend to stretch and widen as you move around.

Note: *Keloid scars,* which are raised and spread into the surrounding normal skin, and are more common in dark skin, require special treatment. If you are prone to keloids, which has a genetic component, you have to be more cautious with piercings, tattoos, surgeries, and injuries to your skin. Treatments are available with the help of a dermatologist. You can't just cut them out, because they can regrow.

Keeping Cancer from Coming Back

Once you've had one skin cancer, your risk of getting another goes up. Don't just cross your fingers.

- Start doing monthly skin self-exams. If you find any marks on your body that you've never noticed before or that look strange, see your dermatologist.
- Set up a series of skin-cancer appointments: If you had a basal or squamous cell, you need to be checked every six months; if you had a melanoma, you should be checked more frequently. Your doctor can tell you exactly how frequently based on your particular situation and the size of your melanoma (for more information, check the American Cancer Society's site at www.cancer.org).
- Speak with your doctor about lowering your odds of a recurrence by starting on a prescription retinoid cream, either Retin-A or Tazorac. These vitamin-A derivatives work deep in the dermis to reverse sun damage, and may stop misguided basal cells and squamous cells from developing into cancer.

If a checkup turns up any *actinic keratoses* (squamous cell precancers) or any seriously sun-damaged skin, be sure you and your doctor talk about the various treatments that can help wipe the slate clean:

- a chemo cream made from the chemotherapy drug 5-fluoruoracil, or 5-FU, which kills off cancer daughter cells
- imiquimod (Aldara), which stimulates immune system cells within the skin
- chemical peel with trichloroacetic acid
- laser resurfacing with a CO_2 laser

- photodynamic therapy (PDT), which uses an acid to target the cancer hot spots, followed by a laser zap

Finally, take stock of your self-care routines. Are you eating plenty of fruits, veggies, grains, and protein? Squeezing in a half hour of exercise every day and seven to eight hours of sleep every night? Practicing deep breathing and progressive relaxation to destress? Using a really protective sunscreen and a UV-blocking hat? Taking care of yourself physically and psychologically has never been more important.

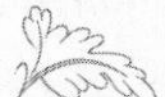

Skin Cancer 101 Here is a brief rundown on each type of skin cancer. They are all on the rise (and the most common of all cancers) thanks to everything from the invention of tanning beds to global warming, which has depleted the upper atmosphere's protective ozone layer. Luckily, a diagnosis of any of these can be treated successfully when found and diagnosed early.

Basal cell carcinoma—the most common and least dangerous

- Typically found on the neck and face, especially the nose.
- What to look for: A persistent, nonhealing sore is a very common sign of an early basal cell carcinoma. Other signs include a reddish patch or irritated area, a shiny bump, a pink growth, or a scarlike spot that is white, yellow or waxy.
- Detected early, most can be treated easily and are not life threatening.

Squamous cell carcinoma—less common but also very treatable

- Can be triggered by both sunlight and bad burns, such as those from scalding water or a fireplace burn.
- Typically found on the head and neck; may also appear in old scars.
- What to look for: *actinic keratoses,* or sun-induced precancerous spots. Squamous cell spots are thick, rough, horny, and shallow when they

develop. You may find that the epidermis is not intact, as there will be a raised border and a crusted surface over a raised, pebbly, granular base. Any bump or open sore in areas of chronic inflammatory skin lesions could also be a sign of this type of cancer.

- Seen two to three times more often in men than in women.
- Most can be treated with little risk of spreading.

Melanoma—the rarest and most life threatening

- Melanomas are black, irregular, asymmetric, growing, and have a rough border. They are especially common on women's legs—it's the second most common cancer in women ages twenty to twenty-nine. Risk rises if a parent or sibling has had it.
- Among African-Americans and some other ethnic groups, most likely to appear in non-sun-exposed areas: on the palms, soles of the feet, mucous membranes, and under fingernails and toenails. (Bob Marley died of melanoma that started on the sole of his foot and spread to his brain.) Melanomas can also form in the eye and the gut.
- If it's detected and treated early, the five-year survival rate is 99 percent. If it's allowed to spread to other places in the body, the survival rate decreases rapidly.

My bottom line: When in doubt, get it checked out. I advise that people start getting annual checks from a qualified dermatologist at age eighteen.

Q: What are the ABCs to identifying skin cancer?

A: First, let me state for the record that I don't like putting the responsibility of knowing what to look for in patients. Being proactive is about scheduling an appointment with a dermatologist if you've never been to one, and being diligent about regular checkups. That said, here is what to look for: funny, changing spots or moles. The ABCDs to check:

- **A**ssymetry—half of the spot doesn't match or look like the other half.
- **B**orders that are irregular—ragged, notched, or blurred around the edges.
- **C**olor changes—say, from tan to black or red to blueish.
- **D**iameter—anything larger than a pencil eraser (6 millimeters) should be scrutinized, in addition to anything that's started growing.

Regardless of these ABCDs, the best piece of advice is this: When in doubt, get it checked out, and visit a dermatologist once a year to have a complete body exam.

10

your guide to more aggressive treatments

Evaluating Your Options and Choosing What's Best for You

As a part-time English professor who lives in a house on several woodland acres in Massachusetts, complete with two ponds and expansive flower beds, Randy sounds like she shouldn't have a care in the world. She has a loving partner, two dogs, and a passion for gardening, a form of outdoor exercise that keeps her in touch with the earth and its rhythms. Her face speaks another story, belying her current lifestyle and making her look older than she really is. That's because most of the damage to her skin was done decades previously and is just now coming to fruition, a kind of unfortunate payback for time spent burning the candle at both ends. Her birthday age is fifty-nine, but her Skin-Age is sixty-five. She exemplifies what's possible on a beauty budget between $500 and $3,000 or more.

In her first appointment with me, I told her that smoking, sun, stress, and sleep deprivation were all major factors in her health, and so are reflected in her skin. She was very open with me about the fact she had smoked for thirty years, before stopping in 2000. "I taught at a school in Massachusetts for eight years that was so understaffed, we had to work almost round the clock to keep it going," she shared. "What kept me going was coffee, cigarettes, and five hours and forty minutes of sleep per night." She knew this figure exactly because her schedule wouldn't let her sleep any longer. Add to that the sun exposure she received from years spent swimming outdoors and the years of gardening, and one can easily explain the lines and wrinkles, the crow's feet, the sagging skin, and the broken capillaries on her nose and cheeks. "My skin is a fairly accurate index of some of my activities," she says. "I was a smoker and a drinker and a person who spent, and still does spend, considerable time outside, all of which don't always register well on one's face. And though I wouldn't call this a high-stress time in my life, like anyone I've experienced relationship breakups, deaths, losses, and disappointments—all of those personal stressors that, if one is lucky enough to have a good long life, one undergoes." Plus, she hasn't had the luxury of a natural peaches-and-cream complexion to hide behind. "Lovely skin doesn't run in my family—it's not one of our genetic strong points," she admits.

So, when Randy walked into my office one day in 2007, she was a virtual canvas of things to fix. After interviewing and examining her, I had plenty of good news: Randy didn't have any suspicious growths or signs of skin cancer, and she seemed to have put all of her unhealthy, beauty-busting habits behind her. Randy gets eight hours of sleep every night and uses sunscreen every day, though I reminded her to apply it to the back of her neck, an area that's vulnerable when gardening. I could sense that she had a good handle on the stress in her life, too—you get better at managing it with experience. It's the stress she has accumulated up to now that has taken a physical toll.

Beauty Alert

The focus should be on aging *healthfully*—not trying to look like a perpetual adolescent.

I started with my usual question, asking what she would like to change about her face, or what bothered her in particular. She gave me *carte blanche*, declaring, "You're the doctor!" Using a mirror in front of her face, I encouraged her to share what she didn't like when she looked in the mirror, and a few specifics came spilling out. "I don't like these marionette lines," referring to the creases from her mouth to chin, "and the fact that I don't have that youthful, wide-eyed look anymore, maybe because the skin on my eyelids droops, making one eye kind of squinty. And there are lots of fine wrinkles on my face, which don't show up in dim light but in good light look all creased, like badly ironed fabric," Randy said.

To help soften the crow's feet under her eyes, the horizontal worry lines on her forehead, and the vertical scowl lines between her brows, we decided to try Botox. This purified form of a muscle-paralyzing substance helps stop the expressive movements that etch in lines and crevices in the first place. Botox can also be used to lift the face in certain places by relaxing the underlying muscles that pull the skin down, which is how I made further improvements. I injected a little Botox into the depressor muscles that drew down the corners of her mouth; to even out her eyelids and make her face symmetrical, I injected Botox in certain spots above her eyebrows. *Everyone's* face is asymmetric, with more muscle movement on one side than the other, and so I adjusted the dose of Botox accordingly, to sculpt and correct while performing the injections.

A different substance was needed to smooth out the lines and folds that ran from her nose to the mouth, and from her mouth to the chin. To bring these creases up to the level of the skin, I injected a filler called Perlane, which contains hyaluronic acid, a natural component of skin that thins as we age. And though Randy was a cosmetic-surgery virgin, she didn't flinch at the needle as it plumped up the lines on her face. Of course it helped that Randy's skin was prepped beforehand with a topical anesthetic, a 30 percent lidocaine cream that I have especially compounded for my patients at a pharmacy. (Compare that to a ready-made tube of what most doctors use, Emla, which contains only 4 percent lidocaine.)

To even out Randy's skin tone and refresh its texture, I painted on a mild 20 percent salicylic acid peel, which removed the top layer of dull, pore-clogging dead skin cells. After three minutes of tingling, the acid self-neutralized, and Randy's face was aglow. To cool things off she was given some ice packs as she left, pressing them to her face as she sat on the train home to Massachusetts. Was she self-conscious? "Not at all," she says, laughing. "There are a lot stranger sights on a train in New York, let me tell you."

About two weeks later, after the slight bruising from the Perlane shots had faded and the flakiness from the peel had cleared, revealing fresh new skin, Randy began the at-home regimen I had prescribed: a twice-weekly application of Renova (tretinoin cream .02 percent) to help treat surface fine lines, wrinkles, and brown spots.

Two months later, in September, Randy returned for a follow-up visit. This time I addressed the redness on Randy's cheeks and nose, wielding a pulse-dye laser called the V-Beam to erase the squiggly little red blood vessels called *telangiectasias*. Randy donned a pair of goggles, held a squishy stress ball in each hand, and listened to me explain what would happen—a sound, a flash, and a pinprick of heat with each zap of the laser. I talked to Randy through the entire procedure, which only took a few minutes.

After the laser work, I took a good long look at Randy's face and decided to inject a little more Perlane in her nose-to-mouth lines and a little more Botox in her crow's feet. Such tweakings and touch-ups are an essential part of the dermatologist's art, as it's safer to undertreat a new patient than overtreat. A few weeks later, after the lasered areas on Randy's face had healed, she was a new woman with a new and improved visage, one that jibed with her inner sense of self. "Even as I've aged, I've always felt young, but lately I'd been looking in the mirror and thinking, 'Oh, my god, is that me?' And now, I look and I think, 'Oh hi! That's me! I look good! I look friendly.'" And while she's happy that the wrinkles are softer and the redness is diminished, she is most pleased that the squinchiness around her eyes is gone. "That's delighted me the most, that my eyes look more symmetrical." The effects are manifold: Because she feels good about the way she looks, she says, she chooses her clothes more carefully, and pays more attention to her hair. "I suddenly want to do everything I can to give myself a good outward appearance."

Randy's partner also thinks she looks wonderful, as do her fellow professors and her students. They have been privy to the transformation, as Randy isn't shy about having had some work done, and has been open from the start to questions from the curious. In fact, she has found herself in the unlikely position of being an authority on cosmetic dermatology, at least in the leafy confines of her college campus. "A woman I work with wants to know everything," Randy says, laughing. "She checks out my face up close every day, watching as the lines disappear. And a retired art history professor came up to me and pointed to his marionette lines, saying, 'I just want to get rid of these; how do I do that?'"

seeking more aggressive skin treatments

It's a given that time, sun damage, and life's highs and lows are transforming your face day by day, even if—lucky you—those changes are still mostly subtle. What's less predictable, and what you'll be zeroing in on here, is how you react to those changes.

When I ask women how they feel about their appearance, what it usually comes down to is: "I'm okay with this, but *not* with this." Maybe the freckle-like spots don't bother them but the spider veins do. Or maybe the uneven skin texture isn't a problem but the deep frown lines are. There's usually a reason. For instance, the spider veins or frown lines may remind them of their mom or grandmother and "That means I'm old."

Another example: I also hear from a lot of women that they are fine with the crow's feet at the corners of their eyes. They'll say, "These are my smile lines and I'd look funny without them. Besides, they come from being happy. I want to keep them." They are part of what I call the physical history of your body, which connects you with your past and who you are. Scars are another example. Sometimes they are a comforting reminder, like a smell or sound, of a specific childhood moment—maybe the day when, after one last crash, you finally learned to ride a two-wheeler. If it's an important memory, you're attached to that scar. It's part of what makes you . . . well, you.

When it comes to aging, where are you on the acceptance spectrum? Maybe you're totally okay with the accumulating lines and wrinkles. Or maybe you want to do everything you possibly can to stop the clock. Or maybe you're somewhere between the two—okay with the crow's feet but not so happy about dull dryness. It's time to figure it out.

how do you feel about looking older?

Let's start with this crucial question, and answer it as honestly as you can: How *do* you feel about looking older? Unconcerned? Unhappy? Ambivalent? Or does the answer depend on what kind of week you've had? Our feelings about our looks are complex, because appearance is so tied into self-identity. Plus, fighting the signs of aging is practically a national pastime. While there's nothing new about this, the pressure to appear youthful is probably more intense today than it's ever been, especially for women. Americans put a premium on looking young and fit. We've even redefined chronologic age, trumpeting sixty as the new fifty, fifty as the new forty, and so on. In the landscape of the forever young, so far no generation—boomer, X, or Y—has escaped the desire to turn back time. And it begins almost before aging starts:

- More than 50 percent of women under thirty in a recent study said they were dissatisfied with their skin, complaining of under-eye bags, fine wrinkles, patchy pigmentation, and other signs of aging.
- In a 2006 survey of women ages thirty-five to sixty-nine, the majority wanted to look thirteen years younger than their actual age! A third said they'd shed six to ten years if they could, and 43 percent wanted to take off eleven to fifteen years.

Admittedly, growing old isn't just fighting off the physical changes, which include everything from stiff joints and receding gums to a slowing metabolism and expanding waistline. There are psychological issues to sort through, too, many of them prompted by changes in your appearance. Take spotting your first gray hairs or realizing that those forehead furrows seem to be permanent. These signs that you won't be young *ad infinitum* can trigger shock, anger, even fear—responses that may be less about a few wrinkles than about coming face-to-face with the idea of growing old.

That's a process everyone has to negotiate eventually, and it can profoundly challenge your sense of self. Even though aging occurs gradually—no one makes a wrinkle in a day—it's not uncommon to look in the mirror one morning and think: Is that me? *Do I really look like that? Help!*

Yet not everyone resents wrinkles. For some, the signs of aging either just aren't that important or are viewed with a kind of pride. (You've heard the words: "I *earned* these lines!") This brings us back to the critical question: Where do *you* fall in the range of reactions, from "Call 911!" to "No biggie"? And are you sure you're being straight with yourself? To find out, try these two quick tests:

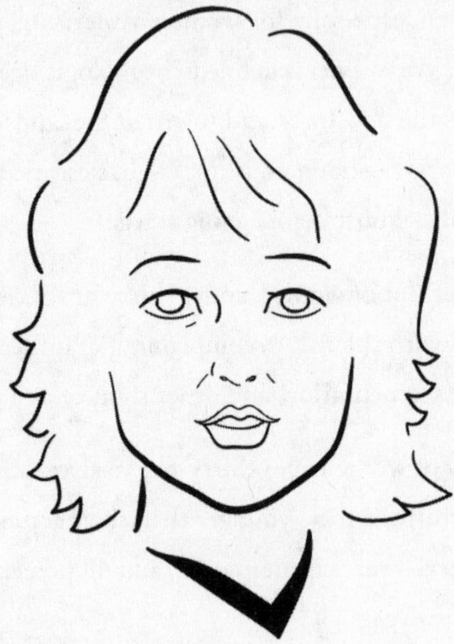

the draw-your-face test—how you look right now

You may have never fancied yourself an artist, but you don't have to be Van Gogh to do this self-portrait. It's fun, and you may be surprised at what you see. Grab a pencil, look in the mirror, and use the blank face to draw in the following:

- Dots for surface skin problems, like brown spots, enlarged pores, redness, acne, ashiness, and roughness (and scars, if you have any, though they may not be age related).

- Squiggles for lines and wrinkles.
- Hatch marks for face-shape things like eye bags, nose bumps, or chin sag.
- Shading for aging you think is stress-related—things that may disappear when you're on vacation, like dark circles, puffiness, and subtle forehead lines.

Note: Just because you have any of these things doesn't mean they're bad, or good, for that matter. Only you know how you feel about time's traces.

Next, use the chart below to do a quick assessment of the things you're okay with and the things that bug you. Score the Not Okay column from 1 to 5, with 1 meaning "Well, I don't love it, but it's not that big a deal," and 5 meaning "I can't stand it and want to change it!"

YOUR FACE SCORECARD: HOW YOU FEEL ABOUT WHAT YOU DREW

FACE AGERS	OKAY Put a check	NOT OKAY Score from 1 to 5 (1 = maybe I can live with it; 5 = gotta go)
1. Fine lines around lips, eyes	☐	________
2. Redness (telangiectasias or small blood vessels) and/or little red dots (cherry angiomas)	☐	________
3. White or brown spots	☐	________
4. Under-eye circles or bags	☐	________
5. Drooping eyelids	☐	________
6. Sagging jaw line/crepey neck	☐	________
7. Frown lines on forehead or mouth corners	☐	________
8. Dry, flaky patches	☐	________
9. Excess facial hair (near lips, on chin, etc.)	☐	________
10. Any changes that remind you of your mom or grandmother!	☐	________

First, look at the 4s and 5s in your Not Okay list; they show you where your age-fighting priorities are. Next, double-check what you're okay with and what you're not, just to be sure you're sure. Three interesting reality checks: Ask yourself if you're doing what author Nora Ephron calls "compensatory dressing," for instance, wearing high turtlenecks or big scarves to hide loose skin on the neck, or contemplating bangs to camouflage forehead furrows. If you could change one thing about yourself, what would that be? What would instantly improve your self-esteem? Finally, here's a critical question: How many of the not okays do you think would improve a lot, maybe even go away, if your life were less stressful?

Guess what? There's a universal answer to number three: Exactly half of the face agers on the list could go *poof*, or at least improve remarkably, if you dial down the stress in your life. They're numbers 1, 4, 5, 7, and 8. What about the other half? What about whatever doesn't completely go poof? For that, you need a little expert help. To find out exactly what kind and how much it costs, keep reading. If you're not interested, you can put this book down now and come back to this chapter later to check in again when you start seeing things you don't like.

what makes you want to change?

If you're still reading, you're thinking seriously about wiping not only the stress aging off your face but going further: investing time and money in prescription lotions and office procedures to erase one or more nonstress face agers. The question is *why*. That's not a silly thing to ask. Beyond eliminating this or that wrinkle, smoothing some rough patches, or simply looking your age (instead of older), it's important to ferret out the *why* because some reasons are psychologically healthier than others—these three, for instance:

- I want to want to look like me again when I look in the mirror.
- I want my face to reflect how I feel: fit, healthy, and younger than my age.

- I'm getting divorced and I need a boost. (In my experience, a do-over of your appearance is actually one of the really positive things you can get out of a divorce; it can be a good first change that often leads to others.)

Here are a few reasons that may lead to disappointment, though not always: Some can go either way.

- My partner wants me to look younger.
- I need to fix my entire life, and my face is the first step. (I call this the Cinderella complex: "Once I get rid of those wrinkles, then I'll get the promotion, win the lottery, save my marriage." Improving self-esteem is one thing, and it can have terrific benefits. But thinking that you'll fix your life by fixing your face, well, no.)
- I need a miracle. I smoked and tanned for fourteen years but now I regret every puff and ray and, oh yes, I'm going to a reunion in two weeks and need to look fab-u-lous. (This kind of external motivator—a reunion, a wedding, wanting to look your best for something special—can be good, but combined with the instant fix requirement, it's a recipe for disappointment. You can do several things that will help but you can't erase fourteen years of skin abuse in two weeks. If only!)
- I get depressed every time I read *Vogue* or watch a Hollywood awards show, and want to do something about it. (The notion that most of us could ever look like a high-fashion model or starlet is, hmmm, misguided. Honestly, in real life, without the magic of lights, cameras, and even Photoshop, most models and starlets don't look nearly as good!)
- I've had five different dermatologists fill this crease/remove this bump—and not one of them has done it right, but I know you will. (Sometimes people obsess about something they see as a huge problem that no one else even notices. It's pretty common and typically starts in the teens. Then it can come and go, flaring with stress: a breakup, a big

move, a new job. The person may get the problem treated repeatedly but never feels better afterward. There's a name for this: body-dysmorphic disorder. It's a condition that typically requires psychotherapy, because it's a mental disorder whereby a person is excessively concerned and preoccupied with a minor defect in his or her appearance. The problem may also be imagined. Without proper therapy, people with this disorder may suffer significant psychological distress that prevents them from taking good care of themselves.

getting real

It's not easy setting healthy expectations for yourself when all you have to do is watch television for two hours to start feeling bad about how you look. Even reality shows are loaded with young, fit women who somehow manage to look good even when they're covered with mosquito bites, haven't slept in four days, and are eating a diet of grubs and coconuts. It's okay to be inspired by the women on television or in magazines, but most of us aren't going to look like that no matter how hard we, or a brilliant skin doc, work. What you see in the media comes with many illusions.

On another note: It's also legit to want to look more youthful if you're in a profession where looks really count, like being a dermatologist! Certain careers (modeling and television, to name two classics) almost require a youthful, high-energy appearance. They are different from law or teaching, where mature looks are viewed as an asset. At the same time, if youthful looks are important to your business life, then fine—as long as it's *your* desire and *your* success strategy that's calling the shots. If your goals are being dictated by someone else or are an attempt to solve a completely different problem, save your money and avoid a letdown. Better yet: Seek some psychological therapy to work out these deeper issues before you do anything else.

Here's another healthy reason to want to update your face: It doesn't reflect you emotionally. For instance, suppose you're as upbeat and energetic as the Energizer bunny but unlucky genes or too much beach time has made you look perpetually tired (dark circles or droopy eyelids) or sad and irritated (downward turns the corners of your mouth, deep creases between the brows). People may avoid including you socially, assuming you're exhausted, depressed, or angry when in fact you're anything but. Time to look into Botox, fillers, and wrinkle reducers? Why not?

Finally, I know of three other positive reasons for tweaking your appearance.

- **Erasing a bit of aging can ratchet up your social confidence.** You know this instinctively, but scientists have actually tested it: Women in one study who, thanks to sun damage, looked older than they actually were felt somewhat anxious and ill at ease. After rejuvenating skin treatments, those insecurities evaporated.
- **People may treat you differently.** Countless studies show that attractive people are more likely to get job offers, promotions, and raises. They're also assumed to be smarter and more competent. And they may even get better medical care—surveys say that, consciously or not, doctors and shrinks prefer to treat attractive patients!
- **It can have a positive domino effect on your health.** When you feel better about how you look, your self-esteem gets a boost, which tends to make you more socially active. I don't mean dancing on tabletops; you don't need to suddenly become the star of the party. However, the more social connections you make and the more good relationships you build, the healthier you'll be, psychologically and physically. And that can be a powerful spark in the drive to do things like eat better and exercise more.

Look again at the things on your Not Okay list, this time focusing on your reasons. Put a star next to the ones that would make you feel genuinely better. Put an *X* next to the ones that are there because someone else is pushing you or that you hope will somehow solve bigger problems at home or work (they won't). Be brutally honest. Changing your looks isn't a cure-all for the rest of your life but it is a great way to feel good about yourself.

what you can do about what's not okay

The nine-day program will make your SkinAge younger and reverse a lot of what bugs you when you look in the mirror. What about the other things on your Not Okay list that you want to change and that you know all the sleep and green tea in the world can't fix? That's where modern medicine comes in, from high-tech moisturizers to smoothing lasers.

There are many skin solutions, some cheap and simple, some not. Undoubtedly, you've heard of many of them, but you may have some misconceptions, too. I'm here to set the record straight so you know what's worth doing and don't get ripped off. First, let's tackle any worries that might hold you back.

Want to Get a Tattoo?

About 24 percent of Americans have at least one tattoo and it's been estimated that up to 50 percent of those people seek to have their tattoos removed. A new technology has just emerged on the market that may be worth considering if you want to get a tattoo, but don't know if you want it forever. A new technique (check out Freedom2Inc.com for information) uses an ink that is encapsulated in microspheres, so the tattoo can then be removed easily with one laser treatment as opposed to current removal techniques such as dermabrasion, surgical excision, and laser surgery.

what's stopping you? the top nine fear factors

If all you've ever done to your face is smooth on moisturizer, suds off makeup, or slap on sunscreen, it can be a little daunting to contemplate injecting Botox, much less much doing more. But fear shouldn't be the thing that stops you in your tracks. A lot of anxieties are really just fear of the unknown, from "Does it hurt?" to "How much will it cost?" So, let's put everything on the table. Knowledge will give you the power to decide.

You're Afraid of Putting Something Foreign in Your Body

Could Botox poison you? Will wrinkle-fillers migrate? Can lasers cause cancer? The answers to all of these worries and more is: no. But in this case, I'm betting a simple no isn't enough and, honestly, it shouldn't be.

- **Botox.** It's made from nasty stuff: botulinum, a nerve toxin that is the most poisonous natural substance known and the cause of deadly botulism (paralytic illness). The Frankensteinian rap Botox has gotten in the media isn't fair. Botox itself is superpurified and actually has been used for more than forty years to treat neurologic and ophthalmologic conditions. It relaxes overactive muscles (that's what makes frown lines vanish). It also resets the muscle balance and lets wrinkles (i.e., cracks in the dermis) heal with the muscles not contracting so hard over them. It must be repeated every four to six months, though, in most people, its effects gradually start to last longer and longer.

- **Hyaluronic acid wrinkle fillers.** Hyaluronic acid (HA) is the stuff in the fillers Restylane, Perlane, and Juvederm, but also found naturally in our bodies. HA oils your joints. HA fillers usually last four to eight months, so you will have to keep going back for more. Concerns that it will migrate—starting out in a wrinkle but shifting elsewhere, creating a lump here or a bump there—are pretty much a nonissue. Bumps can be massaged away.

The rare exceptions can be if too much is put in at once, which is why filling a very deep crease is often done in two steps, if there is pressure on the material—for instance, the very deep crease is under a very big cheek, which presses down on it. Then, there can be migration problems, but they are rare and experienced skin doctors know how to avoid trouble. Even if it does shift, though, it isn't permanent. HA injections last only four to six months.

- **Lasers.** There are lots of different kinds of lasers that can do all sorts of beauty-boosting things for your skin, from vaporizing extra blood vessels and removing unwanted hair to resurfacing your face. What they can't do, fortunately, is set off a flurry of nonstop cell proliferation, that is, cause cancer.

- **Collagen injections.** Because some, not all, collagen is derived from cows, every now and then there's a spate of Internet scare stories about the risk of getting hoof-and-mouth or mad cow disease (BSE) from bovine collagen injections. However, not only is there no real basis for this, but FDA regulations require that bovine collagen for injections come from countries that are free of mad cow disease. Bovine collagen's only true drawback is that it requires a month-long allergy testing process before it can be injected. Fortunately, there are now other types of collagen that contain natural human collagen—Cosmoderm and Cosmoplast—and as such, they don't require allergy testing. These options are purified from dermal tissue grown under controlled laboratory conditions. Cosmoderm is typically used for fine lines such as crow's feet and the fine lines above the lips while Cosmoplast is used in the treatment of deeper lines and furrows, and lip augmentation or plumping.

- **Silicone.** Though not yet FDA approved for wrinkles, medical-grade silicone can be used "off label" and is gaining popularity as a filler because it's permanent: It will finish off a wrinkle once and for all. You should weigh that benefit against the potential side effects: It can cause lasting red, inflamed bumps in some people and, because it is permanent, if you don't like the effect, too bad. Personally, I like silicone for indented scars—it's great to have them permanently gone—but not for wrinkles. To me, there are too many other simpler, safer options. If you like the idea, go only to a silicone specialist, a doctor who loves the material and uses it a ton, because it requires a difficult microdroplet injection technique that takes lots of experience.

A final reassurance: Dermatologists generally use virtually every treatment available not only on themselves but also on their best friends and families, people whose looks and health they would never jeopardize. If you're concerned about an injectible treatment a doctor is suggesting, ask if he or she would use it on him- or herself.

You Think It Will Hurt—a Lot

The reality is that some treatments *do* hurt: Lip-plumping injections, for instance, often elicit white knuckles. Fear can make it all worse, which may account for a lot of the variations in how much true pain different people feel. If you really want to try something and you're really painphobic, try learning some self-hypnosis techniques. (For a site that will give you the basics and lead you to other sites and suggested readings, try www.About.com; then search for "self-hypnosis.") However, there are a slew of simpler ways.

- First off, pain thresholds vary from day to day, especially in women. We're usually most sensitive right around menstruation. So don't schedule treatments just before and during your period.

- When you make the appointment, ask if you can take a painkiller ahead of time. Explain that you're sensitive and scared. The doctor may advise you to take acetaminophen half an hour prior to your visit (but not aspirin or another NSAID, as they may increase bruising).
- When you arrive, ask about numbing agents. These can range from simple ice packs to spray anesthesia, numbing creams, lidocaine, among others. Lots of choices.
- Embrace distractions! They can help more than you'd think. Depending on the person, I give patients a stress ball or two to squeeze, have my assistant hold their hand, use talkesthesia—telling stories, jokes, asking about jobs, kids, vacations, or anything that shifts their attention away from the treatment.

Of course, if you're having something fairly intense done, from laser resurfacing your whole face to filling in multiple deep creases, you're going to need more aggressive pain prevention. This might include a combo of a surface numbing cream, a local anesthetic, and a tranquilizer (often Valium or Ativan) to take the edge off. I also use low lights and soft music to make the treatment room really calming.

The thing to know is this: It all works. During the procedure, you should feel little or nothing, maybe just a faint prick of a needle or a sense of heat or cold or the quick zap of a laser. Afterward, you'll be sore and bruised for a couple of days. Still, if just reading this stops you in your tracks, pay attention! You've answered a key question about yourself: A little, easy-does-it face work may be fine for you but a lot likely will not be.

You're Terrified of Needles

While nobody actually *likes* needles, most of us learn to tolerate them. Not everyone does. If just the sight of a syringe freaks you, this is one fear that's worth working on, and not just to get some wrinkles smoothed out. Life is filled with flu shots, travel vaccinations, tetanus boosters, and more, so learning to help yourself cope can make these encounters easier. The key, again, is to speak up so that your doctor can play a part, for instance, by using the thinnest needle possible (they're easier and faster to slide in).

- Tensed muscles actually make shots hurt more, so while the doctor's getting things ready, dangle your arm to the side, shake it out, and make it as loosey-goosey as possible. It makes a big difference; I do it myself! Or try progressive relaxation: tensing and then relaxing one body part after another from head to toe. Or do deep breathing exercises. (See page 99 for how to's.) Relaxing your muscles eases your nerves and the ouch factor, too.

- Distract yourself. Bring an iPod and listen to some favorite music; close your eyes (so you never even see the needle) and think about something you're really happy about; chatter about a coming trip or a pet's new trick or a great restaurant.

- If you have one, bring a vibrating massager, really! Or ask if your doctor has one. Applying it for a two or three seconds before an injection, an inch or two from the site, is a proven way to reduce needle pain.

You're Worried That You Won't Look Like Yourself Anymore

No one wants duck lips (too much plumper) or a frozen, expressionless face (too much Botox). Sure, there are bad apples in every professional barrel and even in the best hands, complications can occur . . . but they're far less likely in the hands of someone who has a lot of experience. Likewise, good doctors won't make you look like someone else. On the contrary, they'll make you look like you, only younger.

- Finding a doctor you trust will instantly erase a lot of this fear, so do your homework. You want a physician who is board certified in dermatology or plastic surgery. You'll find that some head-and-neck surgeons or ear-nose-and-throat doctors are also board certified in plastic surgery, as are some ophthalmologists who also do eyelifts.

- Schedule a consultation and while you're there, be sure to look at other patients' before-and-after pictures to see if the doctor's aesthetic sense is in tune with yours.

- Take it slowly. Explain that you want to do a little at a time—say, a light acid peel or laser spot treatments to remove red spider veins or dark facial hairs. It's not like getting breast implants, where overnight you might go from an A cup to a D. You can have a little done today and, if you like it, come back in a few weeks for a little more. Do what meshes with your lifestyle, too. If you don't have time (or simply don't want) to keep coming back for appointments, you can choose to get more done at once or stretch it out over time.

You're Afraid That Other People Will Notice

What's the worst thing that can happen? You're sniped at for being superficial because you Botoxed your brows? You feel guilty because a close friend who wants the same thing can't swing it financially? You get compliments and *that* makes you embarrassed?

- First, it will all be forgotten in few hours, as people focus on other things.

- Second, you're simply taking care of your looks, and that's a positive, life-enhancing move. Besides, if you're forty-five but a childhood of oblivious tanning (who knew?) has made your skin look fifty, what's wrong with looking your age?

- Third, you'll be surprised by how many people don't notice. The effect of a little Botox here and some crease filler there may seem powerful to you (good) but the general improvement is hard to pinpoint (also good).

People will just sense that you look better and assume you've been on vacation or tamed your high-stress job or lost a little weight or gotten a better haircut. In fact, I've heard that some plastic surgeons tell self-conscious patients to change their haircut and color because people automatically attribute the improvement to that.

You're Scared of the Cost

Not everything you do will break the bank. A tube of wrinkle-fighting, skin-firming prescription Retin-A may run about seventy-five dollars, for instance, and will easily last three or four months. That's something most people can afford and although it takes two or three months for its smoothing effects to show, patience is your only other investment. On the other hand, some skin treatments are pricey and time consuming. Laser resurfacing can run thousands and take three months to completely heal (though you can go out in public in a week or so with the help of a good cover-up), but the effects last for years. Still, whatever your skin budget is, deciding to spend it can still be unnerving.

- **Do the math.** Divide the price of a treatment you're considering by the number of days it will last to find out the cost per day. For example, wrinkle fillers are usually priced by the syringe (because you can't share them once they're opened). A syringeful of Restylane (hyaluronic acid) goes for about seven hundred dollars and will last at least four months, about 120 days. Divide seven hundred dollars by 120 and you get five dollars and eighty-four cents a day. Now, how does that compare with, say, your daily ration of lattes? Calculating the cost per day gives you a different perspective.
- **Be a smart shopper.** This is simple but important. Go back to your Not Okay list on page 243. Use it to make sure you and your doctor understand what's bothering you most, then explain what your budget is and decide where and whether to skimp or splurge.

- **Charge it.** Almost every dermatologist today takes credit cards and, this may surprise you, there are also finance companies that offer plastic surgery loans. Hmmm. Yes, you're investing in yourself, but unless you're very disciplined you could quickly be facing years of payments and high finance charges. Is it worth the extra dollars and, yes, the stress involved? Think hard about this one.

The point is: Don't be fearful of costs, but do be clear-eyed about them. For some more specific details, see "Dollars and Sense: How Much Does a Wrinkle Cost?" on page 262.

You're Afraid of Looking Bad for a Few Hours/Days/Weeks

Everyone wants instant results and no downtime, but wrinkles aren't formed overnight, and they don't disappear that fast, either. Still, it's amazing what you can do in a couple of weeks. That said, expect anything from pinkness (a lunch-hour light peel or Botox) to some swelling, bruising, and injection marks (a good bit of wrinkle filling and plumping).

- Timing is everything. Don't schedule wrinkle-filling injections for the week of a special event. You will have some bruising (how much varies from person to person) and concealer can only do so much before looking weird itself. Do make filler appointments at day's end so that you can go straight home and apply ice packs to reduce swelling and inflammation. Even better: Take a long weekend, so you've got plenty of recovery time, just in case.
- To minimize bruising, for seven to ten days before and two days afterward, avoid taking
    - aspirin, ibuprofen, and other anti-inflammatory drugs (for minor pain, use acetaminophen *only*). If you're taking daily baby aspirin for cardiac reasons (or Coumadin, Plavix, or Heparin), have your heart and skin doctors talk to each other to work out the correct regimen.

- any individual vitamins, including daily doses of vitamin E and C, which can thin the blood and exacerbate bruising (a daily multivitamin/mineral is okay).
- herbs, especially garlic, gingko biloba, ginseng, and St. John's wort

This is a somewhat cautious list, but why not err on the safe side? Again, it's your face.

- Stock up beforehand on a good concealer to make bruising disappear. I find Laura Mercier's Secret Camouflage is great for covering up small stuff.
- Some laser treatments create eggplant-colored bruises and the only thing that will cover those is DermaBlend (www.dermablend.com). It's been around forever because it does an amazing job. Just get it ahead of time and practice a couple of times to get the hang of blending it.
- If your treatment is more likely to leave redness than anything else (ask your doctor), go to any drugstore and buy a green-tinted concealer; it takes the red out.
- To keep aftereffects like swelling and bruising to a minimum, do the following:
    - avoid strenuous workouts for the first day or two unless you have stitches (say, from a mole removal), then ask your doctor about timing
    - skip wine, beer, and liquor that night to prevent flushing and mild blood thinning (which could increase bruising); underscore this if you're taking painkillers; you don't want them to interact with alcohol

- sleep with your head elevated for a night or two
- scrupulously apply sunscreen, but use a mineral-based titanium or zinc formula to avoid irritation from sunscreen chemicals
- if you're having any kind of skin resurfacing, or a light acid peel, or certain laser treatments (ask your doctor), stop using any skin products that contain retinoids, alpha hydroxy acids (AHAs), and glycolic acids for the day before and a day or two afterward. Again, ask your physician for specific guidelines here.

Treatment Tip

If you carry the herpes virus and experience cold sores on occasion, alert your dermatologist to this so you can plan your treatment around any possible outbreak. Your doctor may advise that you take the antiviral valacyclovir (Valtrex) in advance or reschedule your visit if you already have a cold sore brewing.

You're Scared to Death Something Will Go Wrong

Everyone has heard horror stories about burns, scars, crazy amounts of pain. The most common complications, according to a recent medical survey, are from laser hair removal, chemical peels, and wrinkle-filler injections. The most common cause? Untrained, unqualified practitioners. A growing part of skilled dermatologists' practices involves fixing mistakes made by those others.

- The most important thing you can do is to make sure anyone who treats your skin is properly trained (see "You're worried you won't look like yourself anymore"). Credentials posted on a Web site or even framed on a wall aren't always as impressive as they may look. It's simple and free to find out if MDs are board certified in their specialty, which is the universal gold standard. Go to the American Board of Medical Specialties Web site (www.abms.org) to confirm that a doctor is board certified in dermatology or plastic surgery (or neurology or any other specialty on the planet).

- There are other sites where you can check out specific information about physicians, sometimes for free (www.comparehealth.com), sometimes for a fee (www.healthgrades.com). However, I'm leery of most of them. It's too easy to post misleading information; for instance, healthgrades.com only tells you whether any malpractice suits have been brought against a doctor, not whether the physician won or lost the suit. Imagine if you were unjustly sued and won the case but the only thing anyone knew was that you'd been sued!

Frankly, I'm much more concerned about walk-in plastic-surgery offices in malls that make getting an acid peel or a wrinkle injection seem as easy as buying a T-shirt at The Gap. Not true! I don't think injecting a needle into someone's face should ever be treated that casually.

- Finally, don't let phenomenally low prices anywhere lure you in; they're probably too good to be safe.

You're Afraid That Your Partner/Husband Will Find Out and Have a Fit

Frankly, often men just don't get it. Some see antiaging treatments as frivolous, self-indulgent, or even silly. "You look fine," they'll say. Others worry about side effects or complications, and think what you're doing is dangerous. Still others think it's a one-time event, not something that, like a great haircut, has to be maintained. Finally, some are honestly mystified. If any of this describes your relationship, set up a consultation with a doctor, gather the information so you really know what you're talking about, then decide what to do.

- If your partner's totally, firmly in the frivolous camp, you can quietly go ahead and simply not bring it up again. (But don't pay for it out of a joint account!)
- If your spouse is a worrier, you can also quietly go ahead and see if you get a favorable comment afterward, like, "Honey, you look great!" That's the time to own up and with luck you'll hear: "I guess it's okay, you seem fine."
- If your partner is simply mystified, try talking it out. Explain why you want to do this for yourself, why it's important, why you need his support, even if it's just putting ice packs on some sore spots afterward! Go back to your Face Scorecard and your original reasons for wanting to do this. The better you can articulate it to your partner, the easier it will be to involve him.
- If honesty is paramount and you're both adamant, hold off for a while and revisit it later. At a different time, you both may feel less rigid, and it may no longer seem like such a big deal.

Bottom line: It's your face and your decision, and you have to feel comfortable with it. Only you know what you can/can't live with, and that includes the stress of not telling, telling, or choosing to nix your rejuvenation plans.

Finding the Right Doctor It helps to start with recommendations from friends and family members if you don't already have a dermatologist in mind. Or you can ask your family physician for some leads. What you want to avoid is visiting several dermatologists at once and dishing out multiple consultation fees, so get as much information as you can over the phone before making an appointment. One of the first questions to ask, however, is in which specialty the doctor is board certified. While the prevailing advice says you can go to anyone board certified in dermatology, plastic surgery, or an above-the-neck specialty (such as a head-and-neck surgeon, an ear-nose-and throat-doctor, or an ophthalmologist who has a cosmetic surgery subspecialty), I highly recommend seeing a bona fide dermatologist who specializes in cosmetic procedures first; that is, someone who is expertly trained in this field and who is not simply doing chemical peels and wrinkle fillers on the side. This means you don't want a board certified ob-gyn doing your cosmetic procedure. Should you need the help of an additional set of skills, such as those of a plastic surgeon, your dermatologist can point you in the right direction or work in sync with that doctor.

Also find out which hospital the doctor is affiliated with. He or she should further be a member of a professional medical society, such as the American Academy of Dermatology (www.aad.org) or the American Society of Dermatological Surgery (www.asds-net.org).

Other questions you should ask include:

- How long has the doctor been in practice, and how many procedures like yours has he/she done? Be as specific as possible; if you're interested in getting a wrinkle filler or Botox, ask how many of these the doctor has performed, as well as how many are currently performed daily. You'll want someone who has at least two to three years experience and who performs these procedures frequently. Some dermatologists do not have a big cosmetic medicine practice.
- What kinds of procedures are available to you? Be sure that you have a lot of options, and that the doctor uses a variety of materials. You don't want to be limited.

Your doctor's fees and payment options should also be understood well in advance. As you probably know, elective cosmetic procedures are not covered by health insurance plans.

dollars and sense: how much does a wrinkle cost?

Remember life before Botox? You don't have to go to much further back than that to the days when the most common technique for rejuvenation was a facelift that stretched skin tight enough to iron out folds and crinkles. Unfortunately, the result was too often a caught-in-a-wind tunnel effect. Cosmedicine has come a long way. Today, physicians have the tools to create far more natural improvements without your going anywhere near a scalpel. These wonder workers fall into three categories.

- things we (and sometimes you) can smooth onto the skin (Retin-A, chemical peels)
- things we can inject under the skin (Botox, wrinkle fillers)
- things that create an entirely new skin surface, eliminating problems the first two can't touch (lasers and other tools)

Like most dermatologists, I've developed clear opinions about which treatments I like best for what, but my views are modified all the time to better my individual patient—your skin type, wish list, budget, emotions, time frame, and more.

The three charts that follow give you a quick overview of each treatment category, medically known as *topicals, injectibles,* and *resurfacers,* from what they do best to how much they are going to cost. I've also included some tips on each. Bear in mind that everyone is different and treatments need to be tailored to your particular situation. So if you're thinking about having any of these treatments, use these charts as crib sheets before you talk to a skin doctor or two to figure out what will work best for you. You'll have a far better idea of what they're talking about! Bear in mind that the information in all the upcoming charts can change pretty quickly as new products emerge and old ones are reformulated. Data like this can also depend on several other factors. "Lasting power," for example, can vary tremendously from person to person. Pricing may also entail wide ranges. Use these charts as rough guides. They're meant to give you an overall picture with basic information about these options. For more specifics, speak with your dermatologist.

Things That Get Smoothed onto Your Skin: Prescription and Not

The more researchers learn about the substances (moisture, collagen, acids) that skin loses over time—thanks to stress, sun, pollutants, and more—the better cosmetic chemists get at replenishing these ingredients. Every few months a new hydrating, smoothing, brightening, firming potion debuts. The most dramatic effects come from proven prescription products that speed up cell turnover. There are also some over-the-counter treatments that can help. Here's a chart of my favorites; you'll recognize these because I've already covered them in the book.

PROBLEM	TREATMENT	HOW IT HELPS
Acne Pimples Whiteheads Blackheads	**Benzoyl peroxide** (BPO)	**Kills** acne-causing bacteria; helps control oil.
Acne Pimples Whiteheads Blackheads	**Salicylic acid** (also known as *beta hydroxy acid* or BHA)	**Exfoliates** dead, dry skin cells that can clog pores, inviting breakouts **Calms** inflammation.
Color/texture problems Dull, flaky, oily, or red skin **Texture problems** Dry skin Dull skin	**Alpha hydroxy acids** (AHAs), such as glycolic acid.	**Exfoliates** dead, dry skin cells, smoothing and brightening skin. **Enhances** penetration of other treatments

HOW TO USE IT	INSIDE SCOOP	PRODUCTS I LIKE
If most of face is breaking out, wash with a BPO cleanser once per day (morning, night, or after exercise). **For just the occasional pimple,** spot treat it with BPO cream or gel in the lowest strength that works. Spot treatments are too drying/irritating for the entire face.	**For cleansers,** use the highest strength (up to 10%) you can tolerate without dryness. **Rinse cleansers well** since residues can bleach fabric (clothes, sheets, towels). **To enhance a cleanser's effects,** try using a salicylic acid toner or wash (see below) at another time of day. **For spot treatments,** which are much more drying and irritating because they're left on, start with the lowest concentration (2.5%) and increase strength only if necessary.	**Skin-care counters** Generic BPO wash (2.5%–10%) Neutrogena Clear Pore Cleanser/Mask (3.5%) Topix Benzoyl Peroxide (5%) Wash Clinique Acne Solutions System Neutrogena On-the-Spot Acne Treatment, Vanishing Formula (2.5) **Prescription** Triaz liquid cleanser (6%) Triaz pads (3%, 6%, 9%) Brevoxyl creamy wash (4%, 8%) Duac gel (5% with 1% Clindamycin)
At home, use a salicylic acid wash or toner once a day. **At a doctor's,** a light salicylic peel (20%–30%) may be done every 2 to 4 weeks.	**Start with a 2% wash or toner,** which is actually quite mild. For acne, if that isn't effective in three weeks, try using a BPO wash (see above) at another time of day. **Peels may cause sun sensitivity** making high SPF protection even more essential.	**Skin-care counters** DDF Salicylic Wash (2%) L'Oreal Skin Clearing Foaming Cleanser (2%) Clean and Clear Oil Free Continuous Control Acne Wash (2%) Skin Medica Acne Toner (2%) Stridex pads (2%) Clean and Clear Advantage Acne Spot Treatment (2%)
At home, use products that contain 5%–12% glycolic acid once a day. **At a doctor's,** glycolic acid peels may be done every 2 to 4 weeks using much higher concentrations (30% or more).	**AHA products can be irritating,** even though they're often added to moisturizers. **Start** with a low percentage and work up over time. **If you're using antiacne cleansers,** an AHA moisturizer may be too drying. **AHA treatments and peels** increase sun sensitivity; diligent SPF protection is a must.	**Skin-care counters** Topix Gly Sal 5–2 Pads (glycolic acid 5%, salicylic acid 2%) NeoStrata (physician-dispensed)

PROBLEM	TREATMENT	HOW IT HELPS
Acne Pimples Whiteheads Blackheads **Color/texture problems** Dull, flaky, oily, or red skin Brown spots Fine lines	**Retinol,** a vitamin A-based treatment	**Exfoliates** dry, dead, skin cells, including those within pores, which can make pores appear smaller.
Acne Pimples Whiteheads Blackheads **Sun damage** Fine lines Rough texture **Skin cancer prevention** Basal and squamous cell	**Tretinoin,** a prescription-strength vitamin A derivative	**Has multiple benefits:** It's believed to increase collagen production and decrease collagen breakdown to soften skin and reduce fine wrinkles. Also fights non-melanoma skin cancer and acne.
Acne Pimples Whiteheads Blackheads **Sun damage** Fine lines Rough texture	**Tazarotene,** another prescription-strength vitamin A derivative	**Promotes healthy differentiation of cells** (thereby preventing some skin cancers); treats surface brown spots; helps shed dead cells that could cause acne; acts as an anti-inflammatory effect (so helps prevent flare-ups) Reduces fine wrinkles.
Acne breakouts Pimples Whiteheads Blackheads	**Adapalene** is a topical retinoid that is weaker than others	**Exfoliates** dead, dry skin cells that can clog pores, inviting breakouts.

HOW TO USE IT	INSIDE SCOOP	PRODUCTS I LIKE
Apply to freshly cleansed skin once a day in a serum or cream form.	**Vitamin A** derivatives can be difficult to stabilize, so not all products are effective. **Do not** combine with AHA products—the double-exfoliant action can irritate skin. **Be patient;** it can take up to six months to see benefit. **Slightly** increases sun sensitivity.	**Skin-care counters** Topix Replenix Retinol Smooth Serum 2X, 3X, and 10x (also contains green tea polyphenols) Replinix Retinol Plus
Start by using twice a week at night; gradually increase to daily use. **Apply** to freshly cleansed skin, then, 5 to 15 minutes later, use moisturizer. **Don't push it:** Skin may become somewhat red and irritated for days or weeks before improvement.	**Be patient:** Improvements continue for many months. **Strongly** increases sun sensitivity; diligent SPF use is a must. **Protect** skin from wind and cold, too.	**Prescription only** Renova (0.02% cream) is approved for fine wrinkles Retin-A and Retin-A Micro gels (0.04% to 0.1%) are approved for treating acne.
Start by using twice a week at night; gradually increase to daily use. **Apply** to freshly cleansed skin, then, 5 to 15 minutes later, use moisturizer. **Don't push it:** Skin may become somewhat red and irritated for days or weeks before improvement.	**Available** in gels and creams (0.05%–0.1%), but people with dry or sensitive skin should choose creams, which contain moisturizer. **Strongly** increases sun sensitivity; diligent SPF use is a must. **Protect** skin from wind and cold too.	**Prescription only** Tazorac Avage
Apply to freshly cleansed skin once a day.	**Helps** preteens with early acne. **Helps** prepare skin to tolerate tretinoin. **Increases** sun sensitivity so diligent SPF use is a must.	**Prescription only** Differin Gel (0.1%, 0.3%) Differin (0.1%)

PROBLEM	TREATMENT	HOW IT HELPS
Sun damage Fine lines Uneven pigmentation	**Face creams or serums** containing polyphenols or other skin-protecting antioxidants derived from green tea or coffeeberries	**Two ways:** The antioxidants disarm free radicals that damage skin-cell structures, and seem to stimulate collagen-producing fibroblasts, reducing wrinkling. Also, they may help *prevent* sun damage
Sun damage Brown liver spots Patches of hyperpigmentation (melasma)	**Hydroquinone,** a benzene derivative that fades dark spots	**Bleaches** darkened areas by preventing formation of melanin
Dryness	**Glycerin,** a common moisturizer ingredient	**Both attracts water** and holds it in the skin

HOW TO USE IT	INSIDE SCOOP	PRODUCTS I LIKE
Smear this on at night. Available alone or in combination with other ingredients, such as caffeine, which may enhance absorption.	**Aim high:** It takes a lot of polyphenols to have an effect: look for 90% polyphenols on labels.	**Skin-care counters** Topix Replenix CF Cream or Serum (contains green tea polyphenols) Revale Skin Night Cream (contains coffeeberry)
Apply twice a day and only to hyperpigmented area. **May** be combined with products containing AHAs or salicylic acid.	**Be patient:** Improvements may take 4 to 8 weeks to become apparent. **Stop** immediately if area appears to darken. **Diligent** sun protection is a must to prevent reversal of benefit. **Give** non-Rx forms two months to work; if they're not effective, switch to prescription strength.	**Skin-care counters** La Roche-Posay Biomedic Conditioning Gel (2%) **Prescription** Generic hydroquinone (4%) Tri-Luma (4% hydroquinone, 0.05% tretinoin, and a steroid to counteract irritation) EpiQuin Micro (4% hydroquinone and retinol) Lustra (4%) or Lustra-Ultra (retinol and sunscreen)
Apply twice a day after cleansing and/or using a treatment product such as tretinoin, salicylic acid, or AHAs.	**Look for** a product that also contains silicone for an extrasmooth application.	**Skin-care counters** **Safflower oil** is an effective substitute if acne's no problem. Cetaphil Moisturizing Lotion (but available in *many* face and body moisturizers).

Skin Shots: Things That Are Injected Under Your Skin

Injectible muscle relaxers like Botox and fillers of various kinds may make a face-lift postponable if not completely unnecessary, depending on your preference. Fillers can vastly improve the appearance of scars left by acne or injury, too. There's a menu of safe choices—natural and synthetic, semipermanent (mostly), and permanent—and new injectible materials are coming onto the market every year.

Currently, there are two basic types of injectibles.

- Muscle relaxers (Botox completely dominates this market), which aim to keep frown lines and brow furrows from getting etched in to begin with.

INJECTIBLE	BRAND NAME		COST
MUSCLE RELAXER/WRINKLE SMOOTHER			
Botulinum toxin	Botox Reloxin		About $400 per area, but prices may vary considerably in different areas of the country
WRINKLE FILLER			
Hyaluronic acid	Restylane Perlane Hylaform Hylaform Plus	JuvedermUltra Juvederm Ultra Plus Elevess	$500–$850 per syringe, depending on city
Collagen	Captique Zyderm Zyplast Cosmoderm	Cosmoplast Fascian Cymetra Fat	$400+ per syringe
Synthetic fillers	Radiesse Sculptra Artefill		$850+ per syringe

- Wrinkle fillers (there are several, with new ones appearing every year), which plump up and smooth out deep folds and creases. Fillers can also dramatically improve scars left by acne or injuries.

Which wrinkle filler is used and how often it has to be renewed depends on the location of the fold, groove, or crinkle that bothers you; the effect you want; and the depth of your pockets, since fillers don't come cheap. Doctors almost always make this decision—you're paying for their expertise, artistry, and skill, after all—but it's smart to know in advance what you're getting into.

LASTING POWER	EXTRA TIPS
3 to 6 months; less and less needed over time to maintain smoothing effect.	Headache may follow injection; take aspirin or nonsteroidal anti-inflammatory drug (NSAID) for relief. Have follow-up injection before benefit disappears to maintain smooth appearance.
Typically lasts up to 6 months	Try to avoid aspirin, NSAIDs, gingko, vitamin E, or any other blood thinner for 2 weeks prior to injection. Swelling and bruising is unpredictable, so avoid injections within the week of a major event.
From 2 weeks to 6 months	To minimize swelling and bruising, apply ice to area immediately after injection; repeat every 5–10 minutes as need for 24 hours. Massage filled areas for a few minutes several times a day for 24 hours to prevent bumps.
Radiesse, a year or more; Sculptra may last up to 2 years; Artefill is permanent.	Sculptra lasts longer than other fillers, but filling results may not be apparent for 10–12 weeks. Permanent fillers extremely difficult to remove.

Replacing Your Face's Slipcover: Lasers and Other Resurfacers

Think of your skin as an increasingly well-worn slipcover. Even if you've taken really good care of it, life happens—skin texture will have gotten rougher here, the color uneven there, and it all looks a little dull and drab. Honestly, it needs replacing.

That's exactly what resurfacing techniques do. They remove the old, worn upper layer of skin, and the healing process replaces it with a new layer of fresh, smooth skin. The removal is done with strong lasers, chemicals, or a rapidly rotating wire brush. It's a delicate process, so find an expert in whatever method

TREATMENT	WHAT IT DOES	WHAT IT'S BEST FOR	AVERAGE COST
Ablative techniques	Removes top skin layer. Stimulates new collagen generation in middle layer.	Removing surface problems, such as pigment changes, scars, and fine lines. New collagen creates tightening effect and improves deeper wrinkles.	Average surgeon/physician fees per treatment $2,341-ASAPS[1] $2,236-AAFPRS[2] (includes deep peels, dermabrasion, and laser) $2,160-ASPS[3]
Chemical peel	Depth of peel varies from superficial to deep, depending on concentration, type, and application of acid.	Superficial peels correct minor pigment irregularities and remove dead, dry skin cells. Medium peels improve texture and remove areas of hyperpigmentation, freckles, and sunspots. Deep peels improve wrinkles, furrows, lesions, and pigment irregularities.	$100+ per treatment for superficial peel; $1,000+ for medium depth peel; $2,000+ for deep peel

1 The American Society for Aesthetic Plastic Surgery.
2 American Academyof Facial Plastic and Reconstructive Surgery.
3 American Society of Plastic Surgeons.

suits your needs (consult at least two). How long it takes to recover from the procedure will depend on the size and depth of the treated area. If you have your whole face done, it may take up to several weeks for the redness to go away even once the skin regrowth occurs, but the effect can be remarkable.

Resurfacing your entire face is not always necessary, and spot treatments can also be very effective. Or maybe all you need is a laser that mainly evens out color irregularities, or subtly tightens and refreshes the upper surface. There are lots of options.

NUMBER OF TREATMENTS	RISKS AND RECOVERY TIME	EXTRA TIPS
	Healing time varies depending on technique and depth of resurfacing but typically takes about 10 days for crusting to resolve and new upper layer of skin to form. Redness may take months to entirely disappear. Some risk of infection, pigment changes, and scarring.	Don't underestimate the healing time or the amount of wound care you will have to do during the first week when skin is raw and must be kept moist. Avoiding sun exposure entirely or at least with diligent sun protection using a high SPF, broad-spectrum sunscreen and a large-brimmed hat is essential for several months following treatment.
Superficial peels give best results when repeated every few weeks. Medium peels may be repeated every six months. Deep peels are typically done once, but may be repeated years later.	Superficial peels require no healing time, though skin may be red and itchy for 48 hours. Medium peels cause redness and swelling for about a week. Deep peels create crusting, so careful wound care for the first week is essential. Antibiotics, analgesics, and antiviral drugs are usually prescribed for medium to deep peels. Pinkness may persist for months. Medium to deep peels may cause pigment irregularities and scarring. Infections may occur after a medium to deep peel if wound care is not meticulous.	Medium to deep peels of the entire face are rarely done today because the risks of scarring. Peels of the upper lip can leave a "white" mustache.

TREATMENT	WHAT IT DOES	WHAT IT'S BEST FOR	AVERAGE COST
Dermabrasion	An abrading brush removes superficial to deeper layers of skin. Requires a highly experienced dermatologic surgeon.	Removing superficial and deep wrinkles, texture irregularities, scars, sunspots, and more. Some problems, such as deep scars, can be selectively removed without deeply abrading the entire face.	$1,000–$4,000
Ablative laser	Energy from laser beam vaporizes top skin layers, heats deeper layer to stimulate new collagen growth	Removing superficial wrinkles, scars, pigment irregularities, sunspots, and more. Generation of new collagen has a firming effect so deeper wrinkles and sagging may be improved. Depth of resurfacing can be controlled, varying penetration from superficial to deep.	$1,500–$6,000 per treatment
Nonablative treatment	Varies according to technique used	Removes mild to moderate wrinkling, superficial scars, and pigment irregularities.	$500 per treatment to thousands
Nonablative laser	Energy from laser beam heats middle layers of skin, leaving the top layer intact, which stimulates collagen growth	Improving mild to moderate wrinkling, rough texture and superficial pigment irregularities.	$850+ per treatment

NUMBER OF TREATMENTS	RISKS AND RECOVERY TIME	INSIDE SCOOP
One treatment is usually sufficient for the full face. It may be repeated on smaller areas, such as scarring on the cheeks, after initial healing is complete.	Depending on the depth of the peel, which may vary from one area of the face to another, may take up to 10 days for crusting to resolve. Careful wound care, antibiotics, analgesics, and antiviral drugs are needed after the surgery. Redness, then pinkness, can persist for weeks or months. Some risk of burns, scarring, infection, and pigment changes.	Rarely done because of high level of skill involved. Since it's a very bloody procedure, many doctors choose not to risk HIV transmission from infected patients. Painful, so general anesthesia or sedation plus local anesthesia required. May be best procedure for deep acne scarring.
One	Recovery time varies according to depth of laser penetration. Careful wound care, antibiotics, analgesics, and antiviral drugs are needed after the surgery. Healing is usually well under way at 10 days but redness can persist for weeks and pinkness for months. Makeup can be used after two weeks. Milia (small white bumps) may appear during healing. Some risk of burns, scarring, infection, and pigment changes. Sensitivity to makeup may occur until healing is complete.	Not recommended for darker skin types due to risk of hyperpigmentation. Requires anesthesia. Final results may not be apparent for months.
Most techniques require multiple treatments	No serious downtime; however, various side effects, such as bruising, puffiness, and swelling, may require heavy concealing makeup for a few days. Since deep layers of skin are not involved, risk of scarring, pigment problems, and infection are minimal.	Level of anesthesia varies with the procedure and the person's discomfort threshold. Some require topical anesthetic or local anesthesia.
Three to four treatments over 2 to 3 months	Redness and swelling last a few days. Lesions such as sunspots may form dark crusts before disappearing	Topical anesthetic or local anesthesia to relieve stinging sensation.

TREATMENT	WHAT IT DOES	WHAT IT'S BEST FOR	AVERAGE COST
Intensed pulsed light (photorejuvenation)	Pulses of nonlaser light of varying wave lengths target pigmented skin cells beneath the top layer of skin.	Superficial areas of irregular pigmentation, freckles and sunspots, and acne.	$300–$600 per treatment
Fractional resurfacing (FRAXEL)	A laser beam divided into thousands of pinpoint fractions that vaporize the top and deeper layers of skin, in microscopic dots, called microthermal treatment zones. Skin between zones remains untouched, which is thought to help speed healing.	Fine lines and deeper wrinkles, hyperpigmentation, and scars. Can be used on neck, chest, and hands as well as the face.	$1,000 per treatment
Plasma skin regeneration (Portrait)	Pulses of heat energy directed to superficial and deeper layers of skin where it promotes new collagen growth	Evening out pigment irregularities, improving fine lines, deeper wrinkles, and sagging	$1,000+ per treatment
Light-emitting diode (LED) based therapy	Visible light in different color wavelengths directed at skin surface.	Depending on light (red, blue, yellow, or a combination) is said to improve acne, lines and wrinkles, speed healing, stimulate new collage, improved pigmentation and texture.	$100 per treatment
Radiofrequency (thermage)	Radiofrequency energy heats collagen in skin to stimulate production.	Lines, wrinkles, and sagging skin	$2,500–$5,000 per treatment

NUMBER OF TREATMENTS	RISKS AND RECOVERY TIME	INSIDE SCOOP
4 to 6 sessions, at least 3 weeks apart	Redness and swelling immediately after treatment. Pigment problems, like sun spots and freckles, will become quite dark before disappearing, usually within a week.	Topical anesthetic minimizes discomfort of hot, snapping sensation of light pulses.
3 to 5 sessions, at least 4 days apart	Mild sunburnt look immediately following treatment, and pinkish color that persists for a week. Swelling for 2 to 3 days. Some flaking and possibly crusting during healing. Compete results apparent in 1 to 3 months. Some risk of pigment problems.	Topical anesthetic to relieve prickling sensation. Can be used on darker skin types. Results not as dramatic as ablative laser treatment.
Varies according to amount of energy used: one treatment with high energy or several at medium or low energy	Low-energy treatments require little downtime, though redness may persist for several days. Skin may turn brown and flake for as long as 10 days. A single, high-energy treatment can require up to a week of healing time, during which swelling, peeling, and crusting may occur. Some risk of temporary pigment problems.	Healing is progressive, so skin may continue to improve for a year following treatment. May be uncomfortable for a few hours after treatment. Initial tightness and sensitivity are annoying.
8 to 10 (1 to 2 treatments per week)	None	Painless, but results are negligible and clinical evidence is weak.
1 to 3 treatments every 4 to 6 weeks	Redness, soreness, tingling, and swelling may persist for two days to weeks following treatment. Some risk of burns, blistering, and soreness along the jawline, and scarring.	Topical anesthetic may not ease discomfort. Improvement is mild and unpredictable. Tightening may not be noticeable for six months.

you're not in this alone

Deciding whether to take a more aggressive approach is a personal decision, and one that can take some soul searching. Going into detail about every option out there available to you is beyond the scope of this book. I encourage you to find and consult a trusted doctor in your area so you can have a real conversation about what you may want to consider.

You can also turn to RealAge.com to support your journey, and offer information and guidance in an online format so that you are armed with as much knowledge as possible as you consult with your doctor. The more knowledge you have, the better choices you will make, and the more peace of mind you will achieve.

Don't forget to register at RealAge.com to access all sorts of useful (and fun!) resources. There, you will be able to become a member of our growing community and upload your *before* photo. In addition, the site can help you:

- determine your emotional aging issues
- find a stress and/or beauty buddy
- track your progress
- retake the Happy Skin test when you're ready
- recalculate your SkinAge when it's time . . . and
- post your *after* pics

Plus, I'll be available on the RealAge/SkinAge message boards every week to answer your questions.

Final Note

By now, I hope you've gained not only a lot of information on ways to improve your looks and self-esteem, but also a greater appreciation for your health and happiness, as well as your brain's role in bringing the best of you out. Your beauty is *not* skin deep. Moreover, I applaud you in your decision to take better care of yourself, no matter how small a step you take, starting today. Just picking up this book gives you points! As you no doubt understand through personal experience alone, the way you look says so much about you—your confidence, your courage and character, and even your faith in yourself and the world at large.

Our knowledge about this astonishing link between our brains and beauty will only continue to expand. It is likely that what we discover in the future will reinforce the necessity of honoring time-tested techniques for reducing and managing stress, and choosing to maintain better lifestyles leading to greater longevity. Remember, we want to live healthfully for as long as possible. Looking as naturally beautiful as possible in those later years ain't bad, either.

Your dedication to nurturing your body and skin from the inside out will reward you in so many fantastic ways—not just today, but every day forward for the rest of your life. I wish you the best of luck in your journey and I encourage you to come back to this book when you need reminders about skin-healthy, stress-lowering living. You can go through the nine-day program any time you wish. It might come in handy right before your next reunion. And remember to visit www.RealAge.com for continued support.

APPENDIX A

dos and don'ts for the decades

What You Can Do Now So You Can Do Less Later

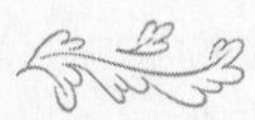

Decade by decade, the effects of stress, the sun, and unhealthy habits will take their toll on your skin. Rest assured that it's never too late to revitalize your looks and begin taking the steps to bring out the most beautiful you.

Here, I'm going to give you the decade-by-decade guide to taking better care of yourself so when you do reach the ripe young age of sixty or seventy or eighty, you can fool your friends because you'll look years younger. The ideas in this appendix reinforce concepts and recommendations already given in the book.

in your roaring twenties

Like any investment, starting early and being consistent earns you the best returns. Now is the time to develop good habits that will protect your skin for a lifetime.

In your twenties, you're faced with the sad reality that it's time to grow up. The decade may bring a host of stresses, from finishing school to starting your first job to coping with your finances to, perhaps, marriage and a family. How you handle them may lay the groundwork for good health and smooth skin, because this is when you must establish and fortify stress-beating coping skills for the rest of your life. It's also essential to learn how to take care of yourself and practice healthy habits because you won't have a parent breathing down your neck or telling you what to do every day.

Don't Succumb to Peer Pressure

One recent government study confirmed that about a third of eighteen- to twenty-four-year-olds smoke and binge drink every month. While that's no shocker, when you add in tanning, often a group behavior learned in this decade, these three vices can do a number on your skin.

You already know what damage the sun can do. Drinking and smoking dehydrate you. Nicotine acts as a diuretic. Cigarettes further dry your skin, making it wrinkled and ashen, while upping your risk of skin cancer. For every decade you smoke, your skin ages fourteen *years*, and not just on your face, but over your whole body. Even secondhand smoke accumulates in your lungs and skin, so watch out for smoke-filled bars.

Do Build Your Social Circle

No one is saying you shouldn't go out and have fun with your friends, but instead of following the herd to Saturday night's beerfest at the local bar and grill every week, try signing up for activities that will actually *benefit* your health. Join sports and activities clubs in your area that will give you options beyond going out drinking. Choose anything you like to do, from hiking to howling to Spinning.

The more you broaden your social horizons, the more options you'll have. The more friends you have, the less likely you'll fall into ruts with the same ones who drink and smoke all the time. What's more, establishing a solid network of friends will help you deal with stressful periods. Support systems are incredibly important in our lives, helping to buffer us against some of the more serious life stresses. It helps to have a variety of support systems, from your academic/school life to your work life, religious life (if you have one), and any other group or community of people with similar interests.

Do Create Good Habits Now

Whether you have habits like smoking, tanning, and drinking to pull back on or not, establishing good habits now will pay dividends throughout the rest of your life. This includes habits like a daily skin regimen and those listed in chapter 4.

Now is the time to begin eating fruits and vegetables more frequently. (How about downing an apple, an orange, or a serving of spinach for every beer you drank on the weekend?) Even though your metabolism might be at an all-time high, you should think about what you are eating and stick to wholesome, nutrient-rich foods and beverages as best as you can.

When outdoors, don't forget the sunscreen, even though you likely don't see any effects of sun yet on your skin. And keep moving; the benefits of exercise are beyond well documented, and your body is in its physical prime to handle the rigors of all kinds of exercise. Gyms can be great, particularly if you find classes you enjoy and keep your workouts fresh. You don't have to be a gym rat or a marathoner. Just put one foot in front of the other and walk, walk, walk, if nothing else.

Do Start Looking for a Good Dermatologist

The next time you visit your family doctor or internist for a checkup, ask for referrals to a few recommended dermatologists, and start your homework. Take the initiative, especially if you've been a sun worshipper and sense trouble in an area, and schedule your first visit with a bona fide dermatologist.

Do Start a Savings Plan

Regularly putting away some of your paycheck every month (particularly if you can do it automatically) can at the very least create a cushion for you for when something goes bump in the night. And you may even be able to start saving for your future (i.e., retirement, your kids' education, your own restaurant), which can reduce stress over the rest of your life. Financial woes plague a lot of people, especially those in their twenties, who may have large student loans to pay off. If you keep a small cushion for yourself, despite your other obligations, it can tremendously help your psyche.

in your juggling thirties

Ironically, this has become the pimples-and-wrinkles decade for many women. Stress, overwork, pregnancy, motherhood, and who knows what else are to blame. Most women find themselves juggling a lot at this stage in life. Plus, the evidence of any bad sun habits start to surface now—fine lines crinkle up around the mouth and eyes, little brown spots may appear on your cheeks or forehead. Cell turnover starts to slow, so your skin may seem a bit duller. Since your DNA repair squad isn't as active as it once was, skin won't heal quite as quickly.

Don't Lose Yourself in Your Life

How can you lose yourself in your life? Try the fifty hours per week that you may be working, and add caring for the kids, cooking, cleaning, shopping, and paying the bills, and it's easy to see how you may have zero time left for yourself. That can lead to stress, physical exhaustion, and even depression.

We all have high expectations of ourselves but, sometimes, you just can't do it all. Beating yourself up over anything you view as your failings won't help you. Neither will missing meals, scarfing down junk food, or skipping exercise when you're stressed. Choose the healthy things you like (walking along the beach, hiking through the woods, going to movies with your kids, planning a special night out with your husband), and zero in on them rather than the negatives.

Do Start Annual Whole-Body Skin Exams

Women in their thirties are getting skin cancer with increasing frequency. Put a note on your calendar to schedule an annual checkup with a dermatologist. To remind yourself, see if you can schedule it the same month as your annual pap smear with your ob-gyn. Make the month your checkup month.

Do Consider a Glycolic or Salicylic Acid peel

It can reverse early signs of aging and reduce acne scarring. How frequently you want to do this, however, will depend on your personal preferences, reaction to the procedure, as well as your wallet. They can add up if you get them monthly but, if you enjoy the effect of a peel, you can do it once every few months and consider it part of your wellness allowance. In other words, don't feel guilty about it! If you have acne, go for the milder salicylic acid peel.

in your new beginnings forties

In your forties you head into perimenopause—the beginning of the hormonal ups and downs that lead to menopause. Wrinkles deepen and skin gets drier and less firm, because estrogen, which maintains collagen and elastin, is on the decline. Shifting levels of estrogen and progesterone can wreak your menstrual cycle, not to mention your psyche.

Midlife does come with its baggage. Those who are not happy with what they have (or have not) accomplished in life may feel on the verge of depression. The forties can be a tough decade, though, and a recent study indicates that anxiety levels and general mental health bottoms out at about age forty-eight and a half around the world (see Middle-Age Misery). The average low point in the U.S. is forty-four and a half (although men apparently continue to spiral until about age fifty-three). The bright side of this decade is that it's often a time for positive new beginnings, too. This is when some women finally decide to stop and take stock of their lives, make a few changes, learn to take better care of themselves, and try new challenges. You know you're not a spring chicken anymore, but you are proud of all your life experiences up to this point and look forward to more.

Don't Get Sandwiched Between Your Kids and Your Parents

In your forties, it's common to feel squeezed between caring for your kids and your aging parents. This double whammy can strain your marriage, finances, and sanity. Don't forget to put yourself first; otherwise you won't be able to help anyone.

Do Double Your Exercise Efforts

Try thirty minutes of exercise every day to release stress. Try yoga, try meditation. You may need them more in this decade than any other.

Middle-Age Misery

A 2008 study that looked at the global prevalence of depression found that men and women in their forties are the most miserable. British and U.S. researchers found that happiness for people in seventy-two countries, ranging from Albania to Zimbabwe, follows a U-shaped curve, where life begins cheerful before turning tough during middle age (no wonder they call it the midlife crisis; this is when you come to terms with your social and economic status, and perhaps have stressors coming from your children and aging parents at the same time), and then returning to the joys of youth in the golden years. Here's the shocker: If you make it to age seventy and are still physically fit, you are on average as happy and mentally healthy as a twenty-year-old.

Do Speak Candidly with your Dermatologist

If you're not happy with what you see in the mirror, it may be time for most aggressive therapies in your dermatologist's office. Don't be afraid, because some of the quick fixes require nothing more than a little prescription cream or the quick pulse of a laser.

in your fine and free fifties

For many women, hitting fifty is a welcome milestone—it's the new thirty. And as the kids start moving out you begin to have the time to really focus more on yourself. It also helps that this decade is characterized by a more balanced state of mind and psychological well-being. You have (hopefully) mastered the art of coping with stress so that it affects you less. You still have to deal with the stress that has taken a slow and steady toll on your looks for the past half a century.

In your fifties, skin thins and the breakdown of collagen weakens elasticity. Most women will reach menopause by fifty-five, leading to permanently lower estrogen levels, less moisture, and drier skin. Brown spots start popping up, and we fall victim to some sagging.

Don't Let Menopause Freak You Out

From hot flashes to mood swings to vaginal dryness to belly flab to erratic sleep, menopause never fails to remind you that there's no turning back from aging. It's also a natural part of a life that all women go through. Be candid not only with your dermatologist at this stage, but also your general practitioner. He or she may have insights that will help you navigate this unique transition.

Don't Give Up on Your Sex Life

There's no reason to let your sex life fizzle. Use vaginal lubricants or moisturizers to ease the dryness caused by estrogen's disappearing act, or ask your gynecologist about an estrogen ring or cream.

Do Consider an Herbal Supplement

If menopausal moodiness and irritability are stressing you out, a combination of black cohosh and St. John's wort, two herbs that have been used and studied a lot in Europe, may help relieve your symptoms. An extra plus: The combo may help raise your good HDL cholesterol a bit. Speak with your doctor before starting a regimen of this combo. In a 2007 study from Germany that showed this herbal combo's positive effects on alleviating menopausal symptoms both physically and psychologically, participants were given two tablets daily, one that contained black cohosh extract and another of St. John's wort. Many reported fewer hot flashes and less sweating, plus a better mood. Again, before adding this supplement, have a conversation with your doctor and get some guidance. Herbal supplements like these do not come without some potential side effects that can conflict with other pharmaceuticals you're currently taking.

Do Increase Your Calcium Intake and Up the Strength Training

Your bones are shrinking (women can lose up to 90 percent of their estrogen, which causes bone mass to drop 2 to 5 percent annually for the five years following menopause). Two ways to help counter this effect and solidify your bones is to shore them up with 1,200 to 1,500 mg of calcium and 800 to 1,000 IU of vitamin D, as well as daily exercise. Strength training in particular is key here to minimizing bone mass loss and staving off bone-thinning osteoporosis. If you were a cardio freak in your younger years, now it's time to embrace more strength training over full-time cardio. Having a few free weights lying near your television or walking shoes isn't a bad idea.

Do Lubricate Your skin with Safflower Oil

Recall what I shared about this kitchen oil: It's high in linoleic acid, a fatty acid that, when you're younger, your skin normally makes to stay moist.

When you're in your fifties, you might need some. Apply sparingly, allow extra time for it to soak into your skin, and prepare to be amazed. In just two weeks, the difference is remarkable.

Do Consider Zapping the Brown Spots

Lasers eradicate them in one to three treatments and religious use of sunscreen can keep them from coming back. Speak with your dermatologist about your options.

in your hanging sixties and beyond

Some people don't slow down a bit in their sixties nor will they entertain retirement. This is the decade when skin surely looks like it's on the downward slide. This can be a decade similar to one's forties and fifties—a time when you certainly don't look as young as you feel. You love hanging out and enjoying life to its fullest, but you don't love the skin that's hanging out all over.

Aging is often synonymous with slowing down, and that's nowhere more true than in the skin's deep layers. Collagen and elastin fibers are renewed more gradually, which invites sagging. Production of glycosaminoglycans—remember those water-loving molecules?—tapers off, meaning skin gets superdry. Skin heals more slowly and there are also fewer immune system Langerhans cells, so skin is more vulnerable to infections.

Don't Go It Alone

Is it surprising that we're back where we started? Keeping up your social networks in your sixties can be just as important as in your twenties. While you probably won't have to worry about peer pressure leading you to the next keg party (then again, who knows?!), a loss of a spouse, an empty nest, or retirement can lead to isolation if you let it. Our number of close friends is declining as it is, down to two confidants in 2005 from three in 1985. And as you get older, you'll not only be facing your own mortality as friends pass away, but gaps in your social structure that you'll have to fill. The solutions are the same as they were in your twenties—stay involved with activities you enjoy that lead to new friends, and keep your social networking going. You're never too old to make new friends and try new things that excite you and keep you feeling young.

Don't Use Abrasive Cleansers or Wash Cloths

Even if you've never had sensitive skin, these days your face can't tolerate roughness, so ban scrubs, cleansing facial squares, and the like. Always use your hands to gently wash your face. Afterward, with your face still damp, apply a creamy moisturizer right up to the edges of your lower lashes (you don't need a separate eye cream).

Do Volunteer

There may be no better way to assuage loneliness and take your mind off your own problems than helping others. And one in three people in their sixties volunteer their time, so you'll have a lot of company.

Do Consider Beating Back That Furrowed Brow

Forehead creases and nose-to-mouth lines can add up to a face that looks unhappy even when you're not. You can try shaping your brow with longer-lasting fillers that erases deep crevices for up to six months. Botox injections can also relax forehead muscles (and, hence furrows) and those in other areas of the face. A brow or an eye lift can also take care of lines and a lifetime worth of sag, pushing off a face-lift (if you were so inclined) for another decade.

By no means is this an exhaustive list, but the more you can keep up good habits through the early decades, the less cosmetic work you'll find you want or need in the later decades, and the better you'll feel year after year.

APPENDIX B:

seven foods that fight slumps

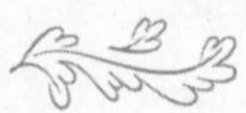

Following are more ideas on foods that can help bust a blue mood.

Watermelon

In addition to the healthy rush of sweetness, you get fiber, a hit of vitamins A and C, lycopene, plus all that fresh, juicy flavor for almost no calories (fewer than fifty per cup). To make your new zip last longer, eat it with some protein and a little fat, as in a fistful of almonds or sunflower seeds, or some low-fat cottage cheese.

A Mexican Baked Potato

Spuds are high on the glycemic index—that is, they give blood sugar a quick boost—which is bad for diabetics but good in moderate doses for other people in need of an energy surge. Potatoes are also an excellent source of vitamin C. Heap on some salsa and top with a dollop of low-fat sour cream to enhance the effect. Spicy foods are stimulating, and hot peppers wake up more than your taste buds. Make it a sweet potato and you get a booster shot of antioxidants.

A Few Dried Dates

They were traditionally used in the Sahara to provide quick energy to camels. Like potatoes, they're a high glycemic snack, but rich in minerals, too, especially potassium. Split the dates and stuff an almond inside for a sweet and chewy candy alternative.

PB&J on Whole Wheat

The all-American sandwich is also an all-round pick-me-up, thanks to its amazingly complete mix of carbs, healthy fats, protein, and whole-grain fiber. Just make it a one-slice foldover to cut the calories down to about 200, and use all-natural peanut butter that has no added sugar or fats. (Look for peanuts and peanuts only in the ingredients!)

Edamame

Soybeans are a top source of *alpha-linolenic acid*, an omega-3 fat that has to come from our diets because our bodies can't produce it. Protein, soluble fiber, magnesium, iron, and folate also make these beans a quick-picker-upper.

Papaya

This is my favorite energy zinger. This bright yellow tropical fruit has fiber and B vitamins; a helpful digestive enzyme, papain, to soothe a stomach that's in knots; and immune-boosting vitamins C and A.

Sunflower Seeds

You'd be hard pressed to find a healthier depression-countering snack than a handful of these seeds. They're fibery, full of vitamin E and selenium for your skin, and B vitamins and magnesium for your mood and nerves. Throw a handful into your next salad.

acknowledgments

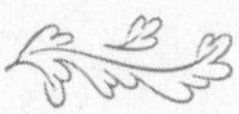

This book reflects the culmination of ideas from a small village of bright, passionate people who offered their guidance, insights, feedback, and, yes, even lots of welcome criticism along the way. I owe everyone a heartfelt thank-you.

First, I give a resounding thanks to my patients who teach me daily about how the body and mind are connected in myriad ways. It's a true privilege to care for them every day.

Many thanks to Kristin Loberg, my genius writer, who digested complicated medical articles with ease, sustained positivity, and humor, and made even the most tedious task a joy. Thanks also to Bonnie Solow who helped bring us together when the book-writing process needed fresh wisdom to keep the goal in plain view and my aim on target.

To the entire group at Free Press (Simon & Schuster) whose support and faith made this book possible. Thanks especially to Dominick Anfuso and his assistant, Leah Miller, and to Martha Levin, Carisa Hays, Heidi Metcalfe, Suzanne Donahue, Eric Fuentecilla, Jennifer Weidman, Phil Metcalf, Barbara Hanson, Laura Davis, Paul O'Halloran, and Ashley Ginter. Thank you to Candice Fuhrman, our outstanding agent.

I am indebted to Val Weaver at RealAge for initiating our collaboration, tirelessly critiquing the manuscript, and being a true friend. Thanks also to other members of the RealAge team, including Charlie Silver, Andy Mikulak, Dianne Lange, Axel Goetz, and the entire research staff. Thank you to Jenny Cook for getting the ball rolling. Thanks also to Dr. Jen Trachtenberg for paving the way for me with her book. And to Michael Black at Black Sun Studio, whose creative brilliance made sure the book met the needs of those who judge a book by its cover!

To Dr. Mehmet Oz and Dr. Michael Roizen, whose support inspires and elevates me, and whose example is one to which I aspire.

Many thanks to my incredible office manager and friend, Melody Cheung, for all of her encouragement and loyal support. Thanks as well to my medical assistant, Ivette Maldonado.

To all of my colleagues and mentors who encouraged me to train in multiple specialties and who have added tremendous value to my practice and my life. To Dr. Alan Shalita for his psychological mindedness and forward thinking. To Dr. Neil Brody, Dr. Michael Jacobs, Dr. Frank Miller, Dr. David Shapiro, Dr. Barbara Landreth, Dr. Chris Creatura, Dr. Ingrid Rosner, Dr. Elliott Hershman, Dr. Orli Etingen, Dr. Richard Fried, Dr. Ralph Lopez, and Dr. Darrick Antell.

To my dear friends who insist I can do anything that I put my mind to. This list includes: Jill Seigerman, Amy Mandelbaum, Julie Berman, Jodie Sperling, Laura Sheehy, Sumeet Bal, Melinda Waskow, Fredda Goldberg, Gabrielle Zilkha, Elizabeth Zoia, Mara Stern Helie, Marcela Speert, Jack Flyer and Winnie Hahn, Charly and Larry Weiss, Annie Partridge, Lisa Gallina, and Andrea O'Brien. To Judy Brooks for making sure that I always have the right outfit for every occasion. To the staff at Kai restaurant and Ito En tea shop for providing a zen environment in which to think. To my amazing lawyer, Marc Chamlin, and to Cathy O'Brien and Courtney O'Neill for handling my PR and marketing so thoughtfully and tactfully.

To the numerous magazine beauty directors and editors who challenge me with their questions, always know about the latest and greatest products, and are priceless sounding boards for my ideas. Special thanks to Ying Chu, Jane Larkworthy, Didi Gluck, Val Monroe, Jen Bially, Cheryl Kramer, Holly Crawford, Eva Chen, Liz Flahive, and Jean Godfrey June.

To my parents, Ellen and Steve Wechsler, who taught me to pursue my dreams and goals without hesitation, and who never doubted my success, even in my lowest moments. To my mom in particular, who knows all too well about the mind-body connection and who has fought with courage and grace.

To my sister, Jodi, and brother-in-law, Jared, for their extreme loyalty and pride in me.

To my husband, Harry, and our children, Zoe and Jaden, who had to deal with the time that this book took from them, and whose excitement and support of this project made it possible.

index

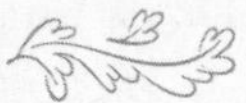

about the author

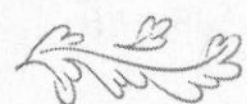

Dr. Amy Wechsler is a member of the American Academy of Dermatology, the American Psychiatric Association, and the Skin Cancer Foundation. A media favorite, often interviewed by *The New York Times; O, the Oprah Magazine; Marie Claire;* and other top publications, she has a unique combination of skills: She is board certified in both dermatology and psychiatry. As a result, she brings an unusually insightful approach to her patients in her Manhattan dermatology practice. Dr. Wechsler graduated magna cum laude, Phi Beta Kappa, with a bachelor's degree in psychology from Duke University. She earned an MD with honors from Cornell University Medical College and completed her residency in psychiatry, followed by a fellowship in child and adolescent psychiatry, and then did a second residency in dermatology. She is affiliated with New York–Presbyterian Hospital/Weill Cornell Medical Center and SUNY Downstate Medical Center. She lives in Manhattan with her husband and two children.